Dietary cholesterol as a cardiac risk factor: myth or reality?

Dietary cholesterol as a cardiac risk factor: myth or reality? was the subject of a scientific meeting organized by the Forum on Food and Health of the Royal Society of Medicine and held at its premises in July 2000. This publication has been made possible by an educational grant from the British Egg Industry Council.

Dietary cholesterol as a cardiac risk factor: myth or reality?

Edited by
Anthony R Leeds and Juliet Gray

SMITH-GORDON
London

Smith-Gordon and Company Limited
13 Shalcomb Street, London SW10 0HZ
Tel: +44 (0)20 7351 7042   Fax: +44 (0)20 7351 1250
e-mail: publisher@smithgordon.com

Available in Japan from:
Nishimura Company Limited
1-754-39 Asahimachi-Dori, Niigata-Shi 950, Japan
Tel: +81 25 223 2388   Fax: +81 25 224 7165

© 2001 Smith-Gordon and Company Limited

First published in Great Britain 2001
Copyright. All rights reserved
Unauthorized duplication contravenes applicable laws.

British Library Cataloguing in Publication Data

A catalogue record of this book is
available from the British Library

ISBN 1-85463-213-2

Typeset by IML Typographers, Birkenhead, Merseyside
Printed in Great Britain by Whitstable Printers Ltd.,Whitstable, Kent

Contents

Preface   7

1   Dietary cholesterol: a review of research and practice over 30 years   11

   Jim Mann
   Departments of Human Nutrition and Medicine, University of Otago, Dunedin, New Zealand

2   Current evidence for effects of dietary cholesterol   17

   Bruce A. Griffin
   Centre for Nutrition and Food Safety, University of Surrey, Guildford, Surrey, UK

3   Genetic influence on cholesterol absorption and its therapeutic consequences   27

   Gilbert R. Thompson
   Emeritus Professor of Clinical Lipidology, Imperial College, London, UK

4   Dietary cholesterol as a cardiac risk factor: current dietetic practice   35

   Gary Frost
   Department of Dietetics, Hammersmith Hospital, London, UK

5   Management of hypercholesterolaemia in primary health care – science into practice   41

   John Ferguson
   Medical Director, Prescription Pricing Authority, Newcastle Upon Tyne, UK

6   Eggs, dietary cholesterol and cardiac risk – a US perspective   53

   Donald J. McNamara
   Egg Nutrition Center, Washington, DC, USA

Discussion   61

Index   69

Preface

The relationship between dietary cholesterol and cardiovascular disease is an area of some confusion. Since the late 1980s, it has been generally accepted that whereas the key dietary recommendation for reducing coronary heart disease risk is a reduction in saturated fatty acid intake, specific advice to reduce dietary cholesterol is unwarranted for most people [1]. Nevertheless, among the general public and even among some health professionals, reduction in dietary cholesterol, specifically from eggs, is still viewed as the appropriate way to reduce blood cholesterol levels. There is also confusion concerning the differences between advice on cholesterol intake given in public health recommendations and that in more specific recommendations for patients with familial dyslipidaemias. Furthermore, although it is now well established that cardiovascular risk is determined by a multitude of interacting risk factors, both modifiable (eg diet, smoking, physical activity) and non-modifiable (eg family history, gender, age), there is a tendency to focus on single simplified messages and to ignore the importance of overall modifications to lifestyle. In order to focus on and to help resolve these issues, a conference was organised by the Royal Society of Medicine Forum on Food and Health in July 2000, chaired by Professor Gilbert Thompson (Emeritus Professor of Clinical Lipidology, Imperial College, London). This publication is based on the proceedings of the meeting.

The idea that dietary cholesterol might play an important role in the aetiology of heart disease dates back to early in the last century, when experimental models of atherosclerosis were developed by feeding cholesterol or cholesterol-rich foods, such as butter, to animals. Subsequently, during the second half of the 20th century, a plethora of epidemiological and clinical studies was undertaken to determine the extent to which dietary cholesterol influenced coronary heart disease. In the first chapter of this publication Professor Jim Mann (Departments of Human Nutrition and Medicine, University of Otago) reviews the key studies carried out prior to 1990.

Both cross-population and longitudinal studies show an association between dietary cholesterol and CHD, but Professor Mann concludes that these studies do not provide strong support that the association is causal. Most likely these results reflect the close association between intakes of dietary cholesterol and saturated fatty acids, which may be found in the same foods. He also points out that the observed blood cholesterol response to dietary cholesterol is accentuated when saturated fatty acid intake is high. Therefore, when saturated fatty acid intake is low, if cholesterol intakes at the upper and lower ends of the usual range of intakes are compared, there is little effect on blood cholesterol. Professor Mann concludes that reducing saturated fatty acid intake is the cornerstone of dietary advice designed to reduce coronary risk and in this context there would appear little need to emphasise dietary cholesterol reduction.

The discovery of the low-density-lipoprotein (LDL) receptor pathway in the late 1970s prompted a series of cholesterol-feeding studies, mainly using eggs as a source of cholesterol, which were designed to establish a quantitative link between dietary and serum cholesterol in humans. In Chapter 2, Dr Bruce Griffin (Centre for Nutrition and Food Safety, School of Biomedical and Life Sciences, University of Surrey) reviews the outcome of these studies and their implications for the dietary guidelines that emerged in the 1990s. He carefully underlines the point, also made in Chapter 1, that these studies used unphysiological intakes of cholesterol (750–1500 mg/day) which, although they resulted in perturbations in LDL metabolism, were of limited value in formulating realistic dietary guidelines.

Dr Griffin also discusses the considerable variation between individuals in the LDL response to dietary cholesterol seen in most studies. The biochemical mechanisms for such susceptibility to increases in dietary cholesterol are believed to include differences in the rate and efficiency of cholesterol absorption from the gut, rates of cholesterol biosynthesis in the liver, the activity of the LDL receptor pathway, and the cholesterol content of bile acids. The variability occurs through the expression of genetic polymorphisms or functionally abnormal genes and Dr Griffin briefly examines the evidence for some of these suggested mechanisms.

Dr Griffin believes that there is an overemphasis on serum cholesterol as a therapeutic target. He points out that the majority of free-living individuals who succumb to premature cardiovascular disease are not at risk from excessively high serum cholesterol levels, but from moderately raised cholesterol levels, co-existing with other risk factors. He highlights the importance of elevated serum triglycerides in this context, concluding that elevated triglycerides represent a significant source of cardiovascular risk that may be modifiable by means of diet, but not by manipulating dietary cholesterol.

The issue of individual and genetically determined variations in the response of serum cholesterol to changes in dietary cholesterol intake, and specifically the factors regulating cholesterol absorption, are considered in more detail by Professor Gilbert Thompson in Chapter 3. Evidence from both animal and human studies suggests that individuals with higher rates of cholesterol synthesis are less efficient absorbers of cholesterol and are less likely to respond to increasing dietary cholesterol intake with increases in serum cholesterol. The precise mechanism by which cholesterol is transported into the intestinal cells during absorption is still uncertain, but several candidate genes have been put forward as possible determinants of genetic variability in cholesterol absorption.

Recent data suggest that an important determinant of the net absorption of cholesterol is the amount which effluxes back into the intestinal lumen. Animal studies have demonstrated that this process is regulated by the ATP-binding cassette transporter 1 gene (ABC1). It is possible that genetic variation in this key regulatory step could explain, at least partially, the observed hypo- and hyper-responses to dietary cholesterol. Professor Thompson suggests that another probable genetic influence is possession of an apoE 4 allele, which is associated with high serum cholesterol concentrations (Chapter 2) and which has been observed to predispose individuals to a failure in response to the statin drugs used to treat hypercholesterolaemia.

It is essential that attempts to reduce serum cholesterol by both dietary and pharmacological approaches are seen in the context of other dietary and lifestyle modification. This is underlined by Dr Gary Frost (Department of Nutrition and Dietetics, Hammersmith Hospital, London) in Chapter 4. Dr Frost reviews the various aspects of dietary risk management as part of overall cardiac risk management where the dietitian works as part of a team, whether in a hospital setting or GP practice, and which aims to improve an individual's risk profile.

Patients frequently present with a constellation of metabolic risk factors in association with raised serum cholesterol levels, including abnormalities in insulin and blood glucose concentrations, low levels of high-density-lipoprotein (HDL) cholesterol, hypertriglyceridaemia, abnormal postprandial lipaemia, hypertension and abnormal clotting factors. This clustering of risk factors has been termed the 'insulin resistance syndrome' and another characteristic factor is upper abdominal obesity. With more than 50% of the UK population now classified as overweight and almost 20% obese, the importance of effective weight management cannot be overemphasised. Dr Frost stresses that recent reports have highlighted the effectiveness of relatively small degrees of weight loss (5% of body weight) in improving cardiovascular risk profile. Such amounts of weight loss represent realistic targets for most people and are more likely to be achieved than the higher targets set in the past.

The approach to dietary advice on fats is also changing, with more advice on individual fatty acids including omega-3 fatty acids derived from fish oils. The role of certain functional foods in the dietary management of cardiovascular disease is now acknowledged, with the acceptance of foods enriched with plant stanols and sterols, which have been shown to achieve a 15-20% reduction in total serum cholesterol levels in randomised controlled trials. Finally, Dr Frost emphasises the need for further research into counselling models that assist people to make the necessary changes in diet and lifestyle.

In Chapter 5, Dr John Ferguson (Medical Director, Prescription Pricing Authority, NHS) discusses the pharmacological management of hypercholesterolaemia in primary health care. In common with the other contributors he believes that there is a danger of focusing on cholesterol because it is a relatively easy risk factor to modify, and, in so doing, to disregard the multifactorial nature of cardiovascular disease. A review of prescribing patterns in England during the 1990s indicates a steady growth in the use of statin drugs, whilst the use of fibrates has remained static. The popularity of the specific statins prescribed has varied with time over the past 5 years. There are also distinct regional variations in statin prescription with a 3.7-fold variation in different health authorities around the country. Dr Ferguson also examines the association between mortality from CHD and statin prescribing across the country, although such comparisons are open to confounding by the recognised geographical variations in CHD mortality, which is higher in Northern regions. He concludes from his data that there was no association between statin spending and heart disease mortality in 1995, but by 1999, there was a closer relationship between the two.

By 1999 there was generally more statin prescribing and the cross-country variation was reduced from 3.7 to 2.6-fold. However there are real concerns that we may be prescribing these drugs at an inappropriate level. Better targeting of statins is required, so that they are prescribed to those people who would benefit most in terms of CHD risk reduction. Dr Ferguson also raises concerns about the risk of treating a biochemical diagnosis, ie a high cholesterol level, rather than treating the underlying disease and re-emphasises the importance of also focusing on other key risk factors, most notably smoking.

Historically, the approach to dietary cholesterol modification, and specifically egg restriction, has been more stringent in the US than in the UK. In Chapter 6 of this book, Dr Donald McNamara (Executive Director of the Egg Nutrition Center, Washington, USA) reviews the changing picture of the scientific evidence over the past three decades and questions the validity of the need for restrictions in egg intake. The persisting recommendation in the US is the restriction of dietary cholesterol intake to 300 mg per day. This recommendation is based on the results from animal studies, epidemiological surveys and clinical feeding trials.

Dr McNamara points out that animal studies are compromised both by species variability in the response to dietary cholesterol and the non-human-like plasma lipoprotein profiles of most animal models. The analysis of epidemiological data using simple correlations suggest that dietary cholesterol is positively related to cardiovascular disease, whereas multiple correlation analyses indicate that dietary cholesterol is not associated with increased cardiovascular risk. Meta-analyses of clinical feeding studies show that the increase in plasma cholesterol in response to a 100 mg change in dietary cholesterol is very small (0.00062 mmol/l). This increase involves an increase in both atherogenic LDL and anti-atherogenic HDL concentrations, with little effect on the LDL: HDL ratio, an accepted determinant of cardiovascular risk. Dr McNamara concludes that available data fail to validate the need for dietary cholesterol restrictions to lower risk of coronary heart disease and reminds us that eggs are low in saturated fatty acids as well as being a valuable source of many essential nutrients.

A summary of the discussion sessions of the conference and the Chairman's summing up is included after Chapter 6. The evidence debated indicates that dietary cholesterol is not a major cause of hypercholesterolaemia or a major contributor of CHD. If people have normal blood cholesterol levels, and are eating a balanced diet, then they need not be concerned about their egg consumption. Nevertheless, in the UK, blood cholesterol level and CHD rates are high and certain caveats are necessary. Firstly, restrictions in saturated fatty acid intake should be encouraged. Secondly, if a person is hypercholesterolaemic they may fall into the category of hyper-responders and at present should continue to restrict egg consumption to 3–4 per week.

Since the conference was held, the American Heart Association [2] has announced that although it will continue to recommend a daily dietary cholesterol intake of 300 mg per day, it has relaxed its recommendations concerning eggs and other high cholesterol foods. It is to be hoped that the outcome of the conference published in this book and the revision in thinking in the US will encourage health professionals in the UK to review their own thinking concerning dietary cholesterol and egg intake in relation to cardiovascular disease.

Dr Anthony Leeds
Dr Juliet Gray   December 2000

References

1 COMA (Committee on Medical Aspects of Food Policy). Nutritional aspects of cardiovascular disease. Department of Health Report on Health and Social Subjects No. 46. London: HMSO, 1994.
2 Krauss RM, Eckel RH, Howard B, Appel LJ, Daniels SR, Deckelbaum RJ, Erdman JW, Kris-Etherton PM, Goldberg IJ, Kotchen TA, Lichtenstein AH, Mitch WE, Mullis R, Robinson K, Wylie-Rosett J, St Jeor S, Suttie J, Tribble DL, Bazzarre TL. AHA dietary guidelines. Circulation 2000:102, 2284–315.

Dietary cholesterol as a cardiac risk factor: myth or reality? Ed Anthony R Leeds, Juliet Gray.
©2001. Smith-Gordon. Printed in UK.

1 Dietary cholesterol: a review of research and practice over 30 years

Jim Mann

Departments of Human Nutrition and Medicine, University of Otago, Dunedin, New Zealand.

Since early in the last century experimental models of atherosclerosis have been developed by feeding either pure cholesterol or cholesterol-rich foods to animals. Furthermore, reducing intakes in experimental animals has been associated with the regression of atherosclerotic lesions. This experimental work has led several distinguished scientists over this period to conclude that cholesterol is a key component of the classical lesion and that dietary cholesterol plays a central role in the aetiology of human, as well as experimental, atherosclerosis [1–3]. This review deals with the epidemiological and clinical research carried out during the second half of the 20th century (but excluding research during the past 10 years which will be discussed in a subsequent contribution) to determine the extent to which dietary cholesterol influences coronary heart disease (CHD), blood lipids and lipoproteins, and other cardiovascular risk factors.

Cross-population studies

Several studies have examined the relationship between dietary cholesterol intake, derived from food balance data, and CHD mortality statistics in a number of countries. Invariably there appears to be a reasonably strong correlation (r usually around 0.6) between these two variables [4]. Similarly, when examining trends in dietary intake and trends in CHD rates a fairly similar correlation emerges [5]. Such associations do not imply causality. Rather, they suggest avenues for further research since dietary cholesterol intake is closely related to many other dietary and socio-economic variables. Under such circumstances neither the dietary nor the statistical methodology is sufficiently powerful to disentangle separate effects. It is quite conceivable that an apparently deleterious effect of dietary cholesterol is in fact due to an excessive intake of saturated fatty acids since both nutrients are frequently found in the same foods.

Longitudinal studies

There is general agreement that prospective observation of individuals whose dietary intake has been assessed and related to subsequent CHD rates provides the most powerful epidemiological means of assessing nutrient-disease relationships. The most frequently

---

Address for correspondence: Professor Jim Mann, Department of Human Nutrition, University of Otago, PO Box 56, Dunedin, New Zealand.

quoted study is the Western Electric Study involving nearly 2000 men from whom detailed dietary data were gathered on two occasions and related to 19-year CHD risk [6]. Dietary cholesterol was reported as being significantly and independently related to CHD to the extent that, based on multiple logistic coefficients, it may be calculated that when men eating 100 mg cholesterol/1000 kcal/day were compared with those eating 300 mg/1000 kcal (approx two egg yolks per day more), the latter group had a 90% greater risk of CHD death. However, when examining CHD rates according to tertiles of dietary cholesterol intake, it is only in the highest tertile of intake that rates are increased. There is no difference in CHD rates amongst individuals in the two lower tertiles. Furthermore when considering the dietary scores of Keys and Hegsted (based on fatty acid intakes as well as dietary cholesterol) a gradient of risk is apparent across the tertiles suggesting that it is difficult to be certain that risk can be ascribed to dietary cholesterol independently of the nature of dietary fat intake.

Three other prospective studies have examined the link between dietary cholesterol and CHD. The Honolulu Heart Program involved the follow-up of 7000 men for whom 24-hour diet recalls were obtained at the initial examination [7]. Dietary cholesterol intake in those who subsequently developed CHD was significantly higher than amongst those who did not, but the dietary methodology employed was relatively insensitive. The Ireland-Boston Diet-Heart Study involved a comparison of brothers who had been born in Ireland and emigrated to Boston (at least 10 years before commencement of the study) with those who had remained in Ireland as well as a third group, unrelated to the brothers, who had been born in Boston of parents who had emigrated from Ireland [8]. While those who subsequently developed CHD had higher intakes of dietary cholesterol than the comparison group, regression analysis suggests that only the Keys and Hegsted scores, saturated fatty acids and dietary fibre, were significant predictors of subsequent CHD. When controlling for the effect of the other factors, dietary cholesterol was not a significant predictor. The Zutphen study involved 857 men born between 1900 and 1919 and who had lived in this Dutch town for at least 5 years when selected to participate in the Dutch component of the Seven Countries Study [9]. The difference in dietary cholesterol intake between the CHD and comparison groups at the time of recruitment (165 mg and 142 mg, respectively) as well as the apparent 80% greater risk associated with an increment in cholesterol intake of 200 mg/1000 kcal [10], did not achieve statistical significance. The conclusions drawn from these epidemiological studies vary amongst reviewers, but in my opinion they do not provide strong support for a causal association between dietary cholesterol and CHD. Rather they suggest to me that the apparent association may result from the fairly close association between intakes of dietary cholesterol and saturated fatty acids, both sets of nutrients being found in many of the same foods.

Dietary cholesterol, blood lipids and lipoproteins

Animal studies have examined the effects of dietary cholesterol on serum lipids and experimental atherosclerosis. Of particular relevance is a series of studies carried out in monkeys by Clarkson and colleagues in the early 1980s. A diet high in cholesterol produced hypercholesterolaemia and lesions comparable with atherosclerosis in humans. At this stage cholesterol intakes were reduced in order to achieve serum cholesterol concentrations of 180–200 mg/100 ml, 201–220 mg/100 ml and above 220 mg/100 ml. After 4 years, monkeys with cholesterol levels in the higher range had very slight regression of coronary lesions and monkeys with serum cholesterol in the lowest ranges had considerable regression [11–14]. There is no doubt that dietary cholesterol can similarly influence levels of blood cholesterol in humans. As early as the mid-1960s it was clear that both dietary fatty acids (saturated versus polyunsaturated) and dietary cholesterol could influence serum cholesterol levels. In 1965 Keys suggested that a 50% decrease in dietary cholesterol would produce an average decrease of about 7 mg/100 ml (about 0.2 mmol/l). He did so when modifying his original formula (ΔChol [mg/100 ml] = 2.74ΔS–1.31ΔP)*, developed to predict change in serum cholesterol according to change in dietary fatty acids, to include the effect of dietary cholesterol (ΔChol [mg/100 ml] = 1.5 [Z_2–Z_1])*. It is important to note that most of the experiments on which the formulae and these conclusions are based involved the contrasting of very high and very low intakes of dietary cholesterol. However, in the light of much research which followed during the next 30 years, it is interesting to note Keys's interpretation of his own data, viz while dietary cholesterol should not be ignored in advice to lower serum cholesterol, attention to this factor rather than the nature of dietary fat is likely to accomplish little [15].

An alternative equation was developed by Hegsted [16], which suggested a rather more marked effect of dietary cholesterol on serum cholesterol than was predicted by the Keys formula. A further important finding to emerge from the Hegsted experiments was that the nature of dietary fat appeared to influence the serum cholesterol response to dietary cholesterol. The effect was more marked when dietary fat was predominantly saturated rather than polyunsaturated, an intermediate effect was noted with monounsaturated fat. Considerable debate followed regarding the importance of dietary cholesterol, with Keys suggesting that the Hegsted equation overestimated its importance [17]. Later observations by Hegsted suggested that when cholesterol intake ranged between 0 and 400 mg/100 kcal daily the relationships between dietary and serum cholesterol was linear but flattened thereafter [18]. Further examination of the Hegsted data suggested that, in the context of a 2500 kcal diet, a change of about 100 mg dietary cholesterol daily was likely to produce a 0.1 mmol/l change in serum cholesterol.

Another major research topic during the 1980s related to the suggestion that some people might respond to a greater extent than others to changes in dietary cholesterol. Katan and colleagues at Wageningen were the first to clearly raise the possibility of hyper-response and hyporesponders to dietary cholesterol [19], though Hegsted had earlier drawn attention to the wide variation in response. The existence of hyper-response was examined by restudying individuals who had shown a 0.5 mmol/l or greater increase in serum cholesterol when changed from a high to a low dietary cholesterol intake and those who had shown no change in their cholesterol level. When rechallenged with appreciable contrasts in dietary cholesterol daily, there was indeed a difference between those who had been defined as hyper- and hyporesponders on the basis of the initial experiment. However, the difference between the two groups was reduced when compared with the first set of experiments [20].

Soon thereafter, our group in Oxford started a series of studies in order to further examine this issue. In particular we wished to examine the effect of dietary cholesterol when contrasting more realistic levels of intake. Most people in Britain and other Western countries consume between 100 and 300 mg/day. Thus contrasting 100 mg with 1 g daily has little practical relevance. Furthermore, since saturated fatty acids appeared to enhance the effect of dietary cholesterol on serum cholesterol, they were themselves far more important as determinants of serum cholesterol than dietary cholesterol, and because reduction in saturated fat is the cornerstone of dietary advice aimed to reduce risk of CHD, we wished to undertake our comparisons against the background of a low-saturated-fat diet. Thus our comparison involved some 180 people (normolipidaemic and hyperlipidaemic) who participated in a cross-over experiment in which they consumed either two or seven eggs weekly. The subjects were all free-living, but consumed a carefully supervised, relatively-low-saturated-fat diet throughout the 4-month study period. The difference between the two and seven egg diets was 0.1 mmol/l which was of borderline statistical significance and questionable clinical relevance [21]. It should also be noted that this was the largest group of individuals to be studied at that stage and, furthermore, that there did not appear to be any appreciable differences in those with normal or elevated lipid levels. The second stage of this research

---

*S = saturated fatty acid intake; P = polyunsaturated fatty acid intake; Z_2,Z_1 = cholesterol intakes on the two different diets.

involved further study of those we defined as potential hyper-responders (ie those whose cholesterol showed a 5% or greater difference when changing from 2–7 eggs) and negligible responders. We then compared the effects of 0 and 9 eggs per week. Negligible responders showed no change at all and potential hyper-responders showed negligible differences which did not achieve statistical significance. Furthermore, there was no meaningful correlation when comparing the cholesterol difference during the first (2 vs 7 eggs) and second (0 vs 9 eggs) experiments [22]. Thus we concluded that when cholesterol intakes at the upper and lower ends of the usual range of intakes are contrasted against the background of the currently recommended cholesterol-lowering diet, there is little effect on plasma cholesterol. Furthermore, under these dietary circumstances there appears to be no evidence for the existence of hyper-responders and hyporesponders.

During the second half of the 1980s a series of further studies produced broadly confirmatory results. For example Hautvast's group from Wageningen contrasted very high and low intakes of dietary cholesterol in the context of high and low intakes of linoleic acid [23,24]. The effect was relatively small on the high-linoleic-acid diet. Another Wageningen study identified people who were defined as high egg consumers (>7 eggs/week) and who were then asked to stop eating eggs [25]. This was associated with a small but significant decline in serum cholesterol, but the contrast was great (200 mg vs 700 mg) and the Dutch participants were following a diet in which saturated fat provided 40% total energy. Porter and colleagues compared the effect of withdrawing eggs in the context of a lower-fat diet and found no significant difference in serum cholesterol under these circumstances [26].

While most of the studies at that stage considered simply the concentration of easily measured lipid fractions as the end-points, a small number of investigators examined cholesterol metabolism on high and low cholesterol intakes using rather more sophisticated methodology. Lewis' group in 1981 compared 1.5 g and 0.75 g added to a diet containing an average amount of cholesterol. In addition to an increase in concentrations of low density lipoprotein (LDL), intermediate density lipoprotein (IDL), high density lipoprotein (HDL) and apolipoprotein (apo) B, there was an increase in cholesterol in the mononuclear cells. There was also suppression of HMGCoA reductase activity and reduction of LDL receptor activity. Inverse correlations were observed between the increase in LDL and HMGCoA reductase activity and LDL receptor activity. Thus they concluded that LDL levels increased on a high-cholesterol diet in those individuals who could not adequately downgrade cholesterol synthesis or increase catabolism [27]. Packard and colleagues in Glasgow examined the effects of adding six eggs per day. In addition to the increased number of cholesterol-containing particles, the researchers found, to their surprise, that the predominant abnormality was an increase in the synthesis rate and, to a lesser extent, a decrease in removal rate of native LDL. Thus, they concluded that those who were unable to compensate were those who showed the most marked elevation of LDL [28]. In his chapter Dr McNamara describes his own elegant experiments which further pursued the mechanisms by which dietary cholesterol influences cholesterol metabolism. However, it is important to emphasise that most of the studies relevant to this consideration were undertaken in the context of a high-saturated-fat diet and with extreme contrasts of dietary cholesterol.

Dietary recommendations

It should be noted that, while most of the experiments undertaken during the period under consideration involved the manipulation of egg intake, for most of the population in Britain (and other similar countries) eggs and egg dishes comprise between one-quarter and one-sixth of total cholesterol intake. Much dietary cholesterol is derived from foods which are also high in saturated fatty acids (eg, high-fat dairy products, fatty meat) so that recommendations to decrease saturated fat intake will almost invariably lead to a reduction in total cholesterol. In view of the clear conclusions from the studies summarised here, that adverse effects of dietary cholesterol are principally evident when comparing very low and very high intakes in the context of relatively high-saturated-fat diets, there would seem to be little need to emphasise dietary cholesterol reduction in dietary recommendations aimed to reduce risk of coronary heart disease. Reducing saturated fat is invariably the cornerstone of such dietary advice and from a practical point of view if there is compliance with this advice, dietary cholesterol is likely to be reduced to levels at which they have little adverse clinical significance. These considerations were behind the rather controversial 1984 COMA recommendations which did not emphasise the need to reduce dietary cholesterol. What advice is now appropriate in the light of more recent research, and in particular the effect of dietary cholesterol on predictors of cardiovascular risk other than lipids and lipoproteins, and the mechanisms which determine their levels in the blood, is a matter for discussion in other chapters of this book and elsewhere.

References

1. Anitschkow N. Experimental arteriosclerosis in animals. In: Arteriosclerosis. Cowdry EV (ed), New York, Macmillan, 1933; 271–322.
2. Leary T. The genesis of atherosclerosis. Arch Pathol Lab Med 1941; 32: 507–55.
3. Wissler RW, Vesselinovitch D. Special lecture: The complementary interaction of epidemiological and experimental animal studies: A key foundation of the preventive effort. Prev Med 1983; 12: 84–99.
4. Stamler J. Population studies. In: Nutrition, lipids and coronary heart disease: a global view. Levy R, Rifkind B, Dennis B, et al (eds), New York, Raven Press, 1979, 25–88.
5. Byington R, Dyer AR, Garside D et al. Recent trends of major coronary risk factors and CHD mortality in the United States and other industrialised countries. In: Proceedings of the conference on the decline in coronary heart disease mortality. Havlik RJ, Feinleib M (eds). US Dept of Health, Education and Welfare, Public Health Service, National Institutes of Health, NIH Publication 79-1610. Washington DC, May 1979, 340–79.
6. Shekelle RB, Shryock AM, Paul O et al. Diet, serum cholesterol and death from coronary heart disease: The Western Electric Study. N Engl J Med 1981; 304: 65–70.
7. McGee D, Reed DM, Yano K et al. Ten-year incidence of coronary heart disease in the Honolulu Heart Program. Am J Epidemiol 1984; 119: 733–41.
8. Kushi LH, Lew RA, Stare FJ et al. Diet and 20-year mortality from coronary heart disease: the Ireland-Boston diet-heart study. N Engl J Med 1985; 312: 811–18.
9. Kromhout D, Coulander C. Diet, prevalence and 10-year mortality from coronary heart disease in 871 middle-aged men: The Zutphen study. Am J Epidemiol 1984; 119: 733–41.
10. Stamler J, Shekelle R. Dietary cholesterol and human coronary heart disease: the epidemic evidence. Arch Pathol Lab Med 1988; 112: 1032–40.
11. Clarkson TB, Lehner NDM, Wagner WD, St Clair RW, Bond MG, Bullock BC. A study of atherosclerosis regression in Macaca mulatta. I. Design of experiment and lesion induction. Exp Mol Pathol 1979; 30: 360–85.
12. Wagner WD, St Clair RW, Clarkson TB, Connor JR. A study of atherosclerosis regression in Macaca mulatta. III. Chemical changes in arteries from animals with atherosclerosis induced for 19 months and regressed for 48 months at plasma cholesterol concentrations of 300 or 200 mg/dl. Am J Pathol 1980; 100: 633–50.
13. Clarkson TB, Bond MG, Bullock BC, Marzetta CA. A study of atherosclerosis regression in Macaca mulatta. IV. Changes in coronary arteries from animals with atherosclerosis induced for 19 months and then regressed for 24 or 48 months at plasma cholesterol concentrations of 300 or 200 mg/dl. Exp Mol Pathol 1981; 34: 345–68.
14. Clarkson TB, Bond MG, Bullock BC, McLaughlin KJ, Sawyer JK. A study of atherosclerosis regression in Macaca mulatta. V. Changes in abdominal aorta and carotid and coronary arteries from animals with atherosclerosis induced for 38 months and then regressed for 24 or 48 months at plasma cholesterol concentrations of 300 or 200 mg/dl. Exp Mol Pathol 1984; 41: 96–118.
15. Keys A, Anderson JT, Grande F. Serum cholesterol response to changes in diet. II The effects of cholesterol in the diet. Metabolism 1965; 14: 759–65.
16. Hegsted DM, McGandy RB, Myers ML, Stare FJ. Quantitative effects of dietary fat on serum cholesterol in man. Am J Clin Nutr 1965; 17: 281–95.
17. Keys A. Serum cholesterol response to dietary cholesterol. Am J Clin Nutr 1984; 40: 351–9.
18. Hegsted DM. Serum-cholesterol response to dietary cholesterol: a re-evaluation. Am J Clin Nutr 1986; 44: 299–305.
19. Katan MB, Beynen AC. Hyperresponse to dietary cholesterol in man. Lancet 1983; 1: 1213.

20 Beynen AC, Katan MB. Reproducibility of the variations between humans in the response of serum cholesterol to cessation of egg consumption. Atherosclerosis 1985; 57: 19–31.
21 Edington J, Geekie M, Carter R, Benfield L, Fisher K, Ball M, Mann J. Effect of dietary cholesterol of plasma cholesterol concentration in subjects following reduced fat, high fibre diet. BMJ 1987; 294: 333–6.
22 Edington J, Geekie M, Carter R, Benfield L, Ball M, Mann J. Serum lipid response to dietary cholesterol in subjects fed a low-fat, high-fiber diet. Am J Clin Nutr 1989; 50: 58–62.
23 Bronsgeest-Schoute DC, Hautvast JGAJ, Hermus RJJ. Dependence of the effects of dietary cholesterol and experimental conditions on serum lipids in man. I Effects of dietary cholesterol in a linoleic acid-rich diet. Am J Clin Nutr 1979; 32: 2183.
24 Bronsgeest-Schoute DC, Hermus RJJ, Dallinga-Thie GM, Hautvast JGAJ. Dependence of the effects of dietary cholesterol and experimental conditions on serum lipids in man. II. Effects of dietary cholesterol in a linoleic acid-poor diet. Am J Clin Nutr 1979; 32: 2188–92.
25 Bronsgeest-Schoute DC, Hermus RJJ, Dallinga-Thie GM, Hautvast JGAJ. Dependence of the effects of dietary cholesterol and experimental conditions on serum lipids in man. III. The effect on serum cholesterol of removal of eggs from the diet of free-living habitually egg-eating people. Am J Clin Nutr 1979; 32: 2193–7.
26 Porter MW, Yamanaka MSW, Carlson SD, Flynn MA. Effect of dietary egg on serum cholesterol and triglyceride of human males. Am J Clin Nutr 1977; 30: 490–95.
27 Mistry P, Miller NE, Laker M, Hazzard WR, Lewis B. Individual variation in the effects of dietary cholesterol of plasma lipoproteins and cellular cholesterol homeostasis in man. J Clin Invest 1981; 67: 493–502.
28 Packard CJ, McKinney L, Carr K, Shepherd J. Cholesterol feeding increases low density lipoprotein synthesis. J Clin Invest 1983; 38: 825–34.

Dietary cholesterol as a cardiac risk factor: myth or reality? Ed Anthony R Leeds, Juliet Gray. ©2001. Smith-Gordon. Printed in UK.

2 Current evidence for effects of dietary cholesterol

Bruce A. Griffin

Centre for Nutrition and Food Safety, University of Surrey, Guildford, Surrey, UK.

There is now convincing evidence to show that dietary cholesterol intakes of between 300–400 mg per day have only minimal effects on serum LDL cholesterol. There is no dose-response relationship between serum LDL and cholesterol intakes because compensatory mechanisms are operative over a normal physiological range. These mechanisms reduce the endogenous synthesis of cholesterol in the liver, activate LDL receptors and decrease cholesterol absorption in the gut. The variable efficiency of these compensatory mechanisms also provides explanation for the variability in response of serum LDL to dietary cholesterol. This occurs through the expression of genetic polymorphisms or functionally abnormal genes which is likely to include those coding for elements of the LDL receptor pathway, specific apoproteins, and enzymes regulating the esterification of cholesterol and production of bile. A genetic predisposition of this kind will be more sensitive to the effects of saturated fat than dietary cholesterol.

Finally, the majority of free-living individuals who succumb to premature cardiovascular disease are not at risk from excessively high serum cholesterol levels but from moderately raised serum cholesterol and triglycerides. The latter represents a significant source of cardiovascular risk which can be modified through diet but not by dietary cholesterol.

Introduction

'It has been stated and denied that diets high in cholesterol result in a significant elevation of serum cholesterol in human subjects', Weinhouse 1943 [1]. Although still worthy of debate today, sufficient evidence has been accrued in the intervening 50 years to qualify this statement and to shed light on the biochemical mechanisms which underlie the variable relationship between dietary and serum cholesterol.

The cholesterol and diet-heart hypotheses

Prospective epidemiological studies in the 1970s established a definitive relationship between serum low-density-lipoprotein (LDL) cholesterol and absolute risk of coronary death which was positive and without threshold [2]. At around the same time, LDL cholesterol was recovered from atherosclerotic plaques in human coronary arteries in amounts directly proportional to levels found circulating in the blood [3]. This evidence

---

Address for correspondence: Dr Bruce A. Griffin, Centre for Nutrition and Food Safety, School of Biomedical and Life Sciences, University of Surrey, Guildford, Surrey, GU2 7XH, UK.

formed the backbone for the 'cholesterol hypothesis' which has now been rigorously tested in randomised clinical intervention trials [4, 5]. These trials provided unequivocal evidence to show that reducing raised serum cholesterol decreases coronary mortality in diseased and non-diseased groups.

The 'diet-heart hypothesis' developed largely from the work of Ancel Keys (as also discussed in Chapter 1) who observed inter-relationships between serum cholesterol, the incidence of heart disease, and diet across seven different countries [6]. Whilst intakes of dietary cholesterol were implicated in the association between serum cholesterol and coronary risk, a much stronger link was shown with cross-cultural differences in energy derived from saturated fat. From these findings, Keys and colleagues were able to formulate equations to predict the effects of dietary saturated and polyunsaturated fats on serum cholesterol. These equations were later modified to accommodate a contribution from dietary cholesterol (Fig. 1). In contrast to the cholesterol hypothesis, the diet-heart hypothesis has not been successfully tested. Review of the literature confirms that the dietary modifications have insufficient impact on serum LDL cholesterol to reduce risk of coronary death [7].

LDL receptor pathway

Perhaps the most crucial piece of scientific evidence to underlie both hypotheses was the discovery of the mechanism by which cells regulate serum LDL levels by co-ordinating the removal of LDL from the blood via the LDL receptor pathway [8]. This pathway consists of a highly sensitive feedback mechanism by which cell membrane receptors specifically bind and internalise LDL by receptor-mediated endocytosis. The activity of this removal process is dependent on the rate of receptor production which in turn is controlled by the level of intracellular free cholesterol. The latter works by modulating the rate of transcription of the LDL receptor gene through the action of nuclear transcription factors known as sterol-regulating binding proteins (SREBPs). An increase in intracellular free cholesterol suppresses the production of LDL receptors and elevates serum LDL, whereas a decrease in free cholesterol stimulates LDL receptor production decreasing serum LDL. A host of genetic and environmental factors exert influence on serum cholesterol through the LDL receptor pathway, mainly in the liver. This includes dietary saturated fats and cholesterol which, as might be expected from their hypercholesterolaemic potential, down-regulate the production of LDL receptors.

The evidence presented so far is incontrovertible but frequently is taken as lending credence to the popular misconception that dietary cholesterol equals serum cholesterol. Evidence to implicate food stuffs rich in cholesterol as causal agents of atherosclerosis goes back to 1913 [9], and cholesterol-rich diets are still used today to induce hypercholesterolaemia and atherosclerosis in experimental animals. However, there is no simple quantitative relationship between cholesterol in food and blood cholesterol. There is a wealth of evidence to show that dietary cholesterol, at physiological intakes between 300 to 400 mg per day, has neglible effects on serum LDL. Moreover, the influence of higher intakes of dietary cholesterol on serum LDL is known to be extremely variable.

Cholesterol-feeding studies

Elucidation of the LDL receptor pathway prompted numerous cholesterol feeding or – to be more accurate – cholesterol-loading studies, which aimed to establish a quantitative link between dietary and serum cholesterol in humans. Since eggs represent the principal source of cholesterol in our diet with a single yolk containing from between 50 to 250 mg of cholesterol, depending on its size, these became the standard dietary format for nearly all studies. Mistry et al [10] showed that the addition to the daily diet of either three

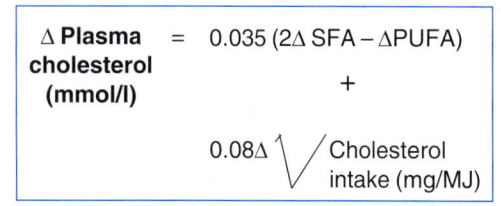

$$\Delta \text{ Plasma cholesterol (mmol/l)} = 0.035 (2\Delta \text{ SFA} - \Delta \text{PUFA}) + 0.08\Delta \sqrt{\text{Cholesterol intake (mg/MJ)}}$$

Figure 1 Equation to predict effects of dietary fat and cholesterol on serum cholesterol [6].

eggs per day for 28 days (750 mg cholesterol) or six eggs per day for 14 days (1500 mg cholesterol) increased plasma LDL cholesterol on average by 15% (+0.42 mmol/l) and 17% (+0.47 mmol/l) respectively in healthy adults. This effect was attributed to a depression in the activity of LDL receptors which was measured in vitro in mononuclear cells isolated from the subjects. Interestingly, the raised dietary cholesterol also stimulated an increase in the concentration of high-density-lipoprotein cholesterol (HDL). This is a frequent finding in response to an increase in dietary saturated fat and cholesterol that contributes to the rise in total serum cholesterol. However, since serum HDL cholesterol is inversely associated with coronary risk and transports cholesterol from tissues, and arterial plaques, back to the liver

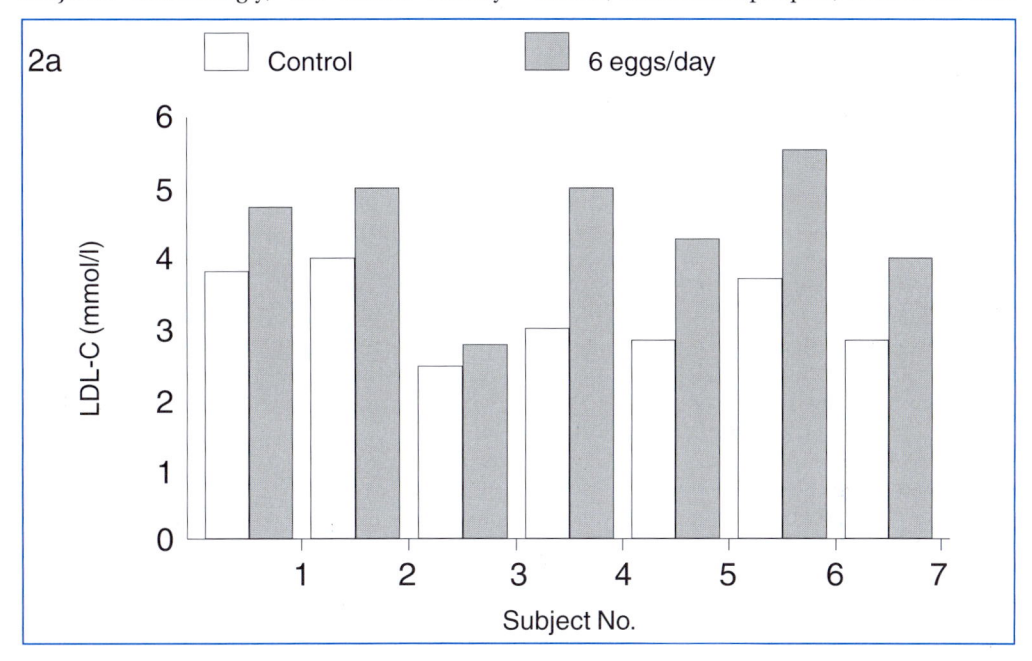

2b		LDL catabolism (pools/day)						LDL synthesis (mg/kg/d)	
	Total		RM		Non-RM				
Con	Fed	Con	Fed	Con	Fed		Con	Fed
0.351	0.317	0.162	0.134	0.188	0.183		13.3	16.4
	$P<0.05$		NS		NS			$P<0.01$

Figure 2a Plasma LDL cholesterol responses to the addition of dietary cholesterol. Figure shows the individual responses of LDL cholesterol of seven normal, healthy subjects to the addition of 1500 mg of cholesterol (6 eggs/day) to a baseline diet for 7 days, as compared to 7 days on the baseline diet alone. Data taken from Packard et al [11].

Figure 2b Kinetic analysis of trace labelled LDL; cholesterol feeding increases LDL synthesis and decreases LDL catabolism. Autologous, native LDL (Receptor-mediated removal RM) and chemically-modified LDL (Non-receptor-mediated removal Non-RM) were trace-labelled with radioactive iodine and re-injected into the subjects. The radioactive decay of these tracers was then monitored ex-vivo to determine the rate of LDL catabolism via receptor and non-receptor-mediated routes, and to estimate of the rate of LDL synthesis. Cholesterol feeding increased the synthesis of LDL and decreased its rate of catabolism principally via LDL receptors (RM). Data taken from Packard et al [11].

for excretion, the increase in HDL is often viewed as a protective response to this change in diet. The metabolic basis for these effects was explored further in vivo in human subjects by Packard et al [11]. This study employed the same dietary protocol, but injected autologous radioactively labelled LDL, some of which had been chemically modified so that it would not bind to the LDL receptor. This novel approach enabled discrimination between LDL that was catabolised by LDL receptors or by non-receptor-mediated pathways. The addition of six eggs a day to a background diet again elevated serum LDL cholesterol (+40%) (Fig. 2a) and also HDL cholesterol (+18%). The increase in LDL was ascribed to an increase in the number of LDL particles and not to a change in the composition of LDL. The catabolism of LDL, via LDL receptors, and LDL synthesis were shown to be decreased and increased respectively (Fig. 2b). Despite an overall decrease in LDL catabolism, in absolute terms, more LDL was removed by non-receptor or scavenger pathways, a route of catabolism considered to be more atherogenic.

Changing views: 1994 to 1997

Guideline statements on the effects of dietary cholesterol on serum cholesterol produced by the Committee for Medical Aspects of Food (COMA) were clearly influenced by these early cholesterol-feeding studies and in 1994 reported: 'The weight of evidence supports the view that raising dietary cholesterol increases serum cholesterol, although there is considerable inter-individual variation' [12]. The outcome of such statements was to recommend that dietary cholesterol intakes in the UK should not rise above 250 mg per day. An inherent problem with this and other more extreme recommendations is that they were derived from studies which used unphysiological intakes of cholesterol (750–1500 mg/day). These intakes were extreme for the chief purpose of perturbing LDL metabolism and, though informative, were of limited practical value for formulating dietary guidelines. In particular, compliance with these recommendations meant virtually excluding eggs from the diet. This problem was addressed in subsequent studies which focused on the effects of more physiological intakes of dietary cholesterol. These studies confirmed the lack of a dose-response relationship between dietary and serum cholesterol over a range of cholesterol intakes between 80 to 850 mg per day. With the notable exception of studies which included a concomitant increase in saturated fat, all showed that dietary cholesterol produces only minimal effects on serum cholesterol (Table 1). These findings prompted clarification of the earlier statement from the COMA panel which in 1991 reported that: 'Dietary cholesterol intake has a small effect on serum cholesterol levels' [13]. They also made it possible to define with greater accuracy the serum cholesterol response to a standard daily intake of dietary cholesterol. For example, an increase in dietary cholesterol of 100 mg should elicit an average increase in serum cholesterol of between 0.10 to 0.13 mmol/l [14]. Whereas the equations of

Table 1 Cholesterol-feeding studies between 1994 and 1999. Intakes of dietary cholesterol between 80 to 858 mg per day for up to 8 weeks produced minimal increases in LDL cholesterol in normal healthy male (M) and females (F), vegetarians (veg), females with gallstones (F gall) and hyperlipidaemic subjects (Hyper-Lp). Studies which included an increase in saturated fat (+SFA) showed markedly greater increases in LDL cholesterol.

Author	Year	[Ref]	Subjects (n)	Duration (weeks)	Dose (mg/d)	Δ Plasma cholesterol (mmol/l per 100 mg/d)
Ginsberg	1994	[25]	M (24)	8	128–858	0.04
Schnohr	1994	[26]	M/F (24)	6	230	0.06
Vuoristo	1994	[27]	Veg (5)	8	690	0.09
Kern	1994	[28]	F gall (16)	3	939	0.02
Ginsberg	1995	[29]	F (13)	8	128–690	0.07
Knopp	1996	[30]	HyperLp (75)	8	128–468	0.08
Sehayek	1998	[16]	M/F (18)	3	80–200	0.30 (+SFA)
Clifton	1998	[31]	M/F (105)	3	650–840	0.29 (+SFA)

Keys would agree with this value in most situations, examination of the data in Table 1 would indicate even this to be an over-estimate. In considering the practical application of these consensus values, it is important to appreciate the following. First, saturated fat will exert a greater influence on serum cholesterol than dietary cholesterol simply by virtue of its greater abundance in the diet. Second, if an average egg yolk contains 150 mg of cholesterol, the daily addition of one, or occasionally two, eggs to a diet is going to have no significant impact on serum LDL cholesterol.

Mechanisms to explain hyper and hyporesponders to dietary cholesterol

Nearly all studies performed to date show considerable inter-individual variation in the LDL response to dietary cholesterol. An estimated figure for the proportion of individuals who may be more responsive to dietary cholesterol is about 20% of populations studied to date, though this figure has yet to be confirmed. The biochemical mechanisms which may render an individual either more or less susceptible to the hypercholesterolaemic effects of dietary cholesterol have been identified. These may include differences in the rate and efficiency of cholesterol absorption in the gut, rates of cholesterol biosynthesis in the liver, the activity of the LDL receptor pathway, and the cholesterol content of bile acids. These processes are interrelated, such that an aberration in one is very likely to affect the others. The liver compensates for increases in dietary cholesterol over a physiological range by shutting down endogenous cholesterol synthesis, and the sensitivity of this mechanism may contribute to inter-individual variation in the response of serum LDL. There is also evidence to implicate the absorption of dietary cholesterol as a compensatory mechanism for increasing levels of dietary intake, though whether this is linked to the variation in LDL response is not clear.

It is well established that unphysiologically-high levels of dietary cholesterol intake (>750 mg/day) shut down cholesterol absorption in the gut and that the absorption of cholesterol

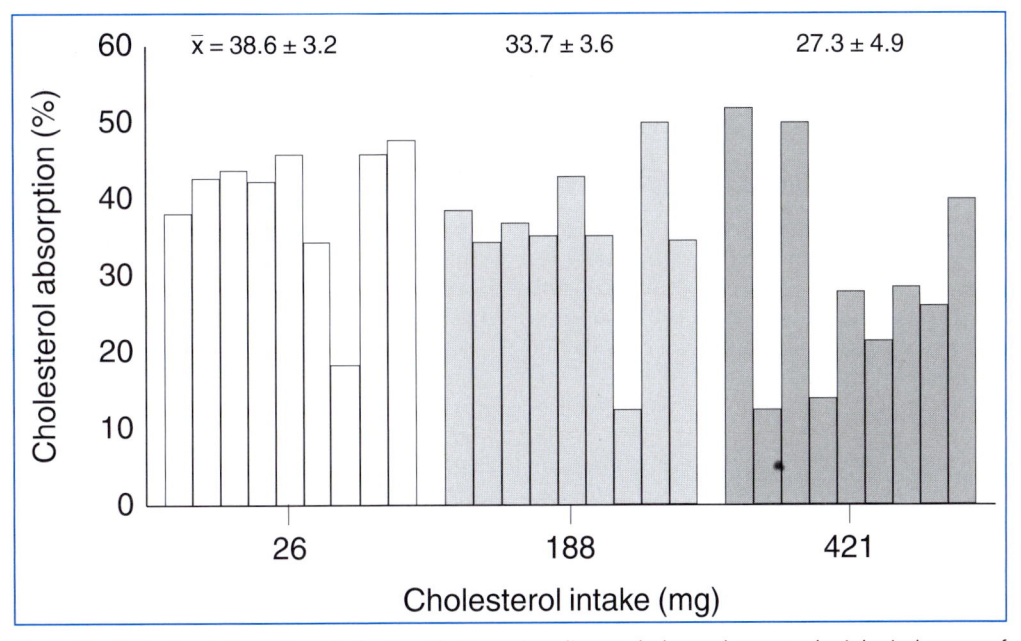

Figure 3 Cholesterol absorption declines with increasing dietary cholesterol over a physiological range of intakes. Individual and mean percentage absorption of dietary cholesterol are shown, as measured by mass spectrometry at high (421 mg/day) and low (188 mg/day) acute doses of cholesterol intake. Pentadeuterated cholesterol (26 mg) was given as the tracer at high and low doses of natural cholesterol, and also in the absence of cholesterol. There was a general diminution of response from low-to-high cholesterol intakes and a five-fold variation in response at the high level of intake. Data taken from Ostlund et al [15].

in the gut is inversely proportion to the biosynthesis of cholesterol in the liver. The possibility of a dose-response relationship existing between these parameters at lower levels of cholesterol intake was recently examined by Ostlund et al [15]. Their study revealed that cholesterol absorption actually decreases over a normal physiological range (21–421 mg/day). Cholesterol absorption markedly declined in some individuals at the upper level which may have represented a threshold value in these subjects, though there was still a five-fold difference in percentage absorption between subjects at this level of intake (Fig. 3). No relationship could be found between cholesterol absorption and changes in serum LDL across this range of cholesterol intakes. In an earlier study, Sehayek et al [16] also examined the relationship between cholesterol absorption and serum LDL. In accord with the previous study, there was no relationship between the percentage of cholesterol absorbed with serum LDL or HDL cholesterol. However, analysis of the relative change in these paremeters revealed an interesting pattern of results which may provide clues as to the source of inter-individual variation in dietary response. The change in percentage of cholesterol absorption on a high-fat (43% fat, 44% saturated), high-cholesterol (range 460–700 mg/day) diet relative to a high-fat, low-cholesterol (range 184–280 mg) diet was shown to account for two-thirds of the variability in serum LDL levels (r^2 = 62% P<0.005) and a lesser but still significant proportion of variability in HDL (r^2 = 48% P<0.05). In addition, the change in cholesterol absorption showed a 'U-shape' relationship with the changes in serum LDL and HDL identifying two groups of patients who showed increases in LDL-cholesterol of around 20%, in the main, but changes in cholesterol absorption ranging between –10% to +10%. This finding raised the intriguing question as to why dietary cholesterol should exert opposite effects on cholesterol absorption and yet produce the same effect on serum LDL? The explanation given considers the relationship between the composition of bile and cholesterol absorption. Bile contains bile acids and phospholipids which are required to solubilise fat to faciliate its absorption in the gut.

Bile also contains free cholesterol, the concentration of which is inversely related to cholesterol absorption through competition with dietary cholesterol. The authors proposed that genetic differences in the rate-limiting enzyme for bile acid production from cholesterol in the liver, 7-α-hydroxylase, may account for this variability through influencing the relative proportion of cholesterol to bile acids and phospholipids. How this explains the variability in serum LDL is still not clear but is likely to involve a complex interplay between cholesterol biosynthesis, intracellular free cholesterol and control of the LDL receptor pathway.

Effects of dietary cholesterol on serum LDL are modulated by apo E-phenotype

Apoprotein E (apo E) is a constituent of lipoproteins which acts as major ligand for binding triglyceride-rich lipoproteins and their remnants to the LDL receptor and to a closely related receptor known as the remnant receptor. The gene that codes for apo E is polymorphic and gives rise to three different but commonly occurring isoforms of the apoprotein, namely E2, E3 and E4, which bind to the receptor with increasing affinity in the order E2>E3>E4. For a full review see Wu et al [17]. The apo E polymorphism has been reported to account for up to 8% of variation in serum LDL cholesterol levels in populations. Carriers of E4 and E2 show higher and lower than average concentrations of serum LDL cholesterol respectively as a result of differential effects of these isoforms on the activity of LDL receptors. This finding has been associated with increased cardiovascular risk in the former group and an impaired capacity to remove triglyceride-rich lipoproteins in the latter. The relevance of this effect in the present context is that carriers of apo E4 show increased sensitivity to dietary fats and dietary cholesterol with respect to an increase in serum LDL. One predisposing factor for this effect is thought to be the down-regulation of the LDL receptor pathway as a result of the relatively greater receptor-mediated uptake of lipoproteins which effectively increases free cholesterol within the cell. An alternative, though not necessarily unrelated explanation, comes from

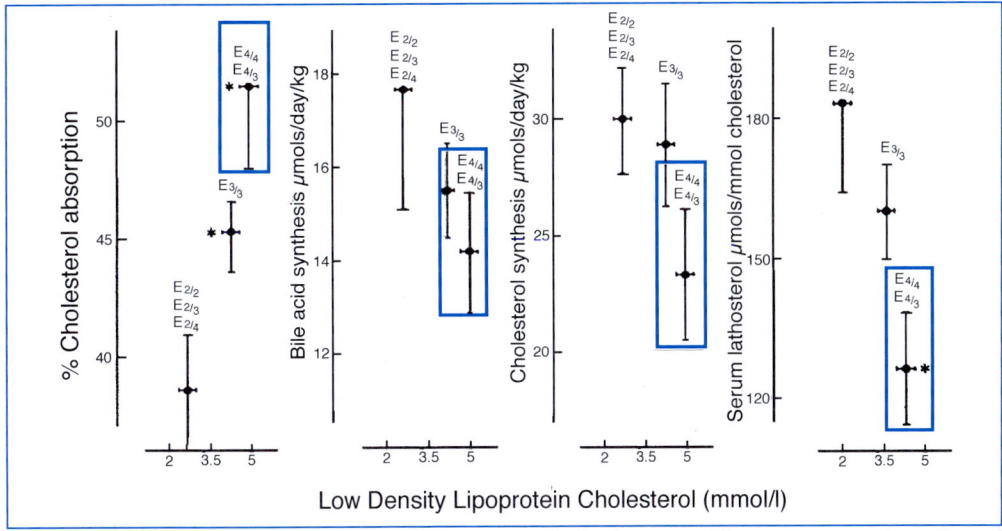

Figure 4 Cholesterol absorption is related to apoprotein E phenotype. The percentage absorption of cholesterol was measured in 300 men on a habitual diet over 7 days by the difference between a dose of radioactively-labelled dietary cholesterol and that recovered in faeces as bile acids and neutral sterols. Subjects carrying apo E4 (E4/E4, E4/E3) showed the highest LDL cholesterol and percentage cholesterol absorption, and the lowest production of bile acids and endogenous synthesis of cholesterol as compared to other E phenotypes. Data taken from Kesaniemi et al [18].

the observation that E4 carriers absorb dietary cholesterol more efficiently than carriers of E2 or E3 [18]. The reciprocal relationship between the absorption and biosynthesis of cholesterol means that carriers of E4 are naturally low synthesizers of cholesterol. (Note that the enhanced uptake of circulating cholesterol would also down regulate cholesterol synthesis in the cell). In the same study, carriers of apo E4 were also shown to produce less bile acids than their counterparts (Fig. 4). Although this study did not examine the effects of increasing dietary cholesterol or the composition of bile, this finding would appear to be at odds with the more efficient absorption of cholesterol and suggests that apo E4 in some way facilitates the production and transport of dietary cholesterol in chylomicrons. This may accelerate the flux of cholesterol into and across the enterocyte but would be independent of micelle formation and the production of bile acids. Whatever the biochemical mechanism, the frequency of apo E4 can be as high as 20% in northern Europeans and even higher amongst selected, free-living dyslipidaemic groups. Whilst these individuals may show increased susceptibility to dietary cholesterol, they may be equally more responsive to reductions in dietary fat and to modifications in the type of dietary polyunsaturated fat. It is possible that these potentially beneficial changes in the amount and type of fat will outweigh the adverse effects of dietary cholesterol in this group. Apo E phenotype may therefore play a role in modulating the LDL response to dietary cholesterol, though its contribution as a major factor to variation in serum LDL levels has been recently challenged by Glatz et al [19].

Serum cholesterol and triglycerides as cardiac risk factors within populations

As previously discussed, the absolute risk associated with serum cholesterol and the reduction in this risk in clinical trials is beyond dispute. However, the cholesterol hypothesis provides an inadequate basis on which to explain the effects of diet on cardiovascular risk. This is particularly evident from the failure of dietary intervention trials to decrease coronary mortality, principally because they were been unable to achieve reductions in serum LDL commensurate with that of the cholesterol-lowering drugs. Whilst the generally poor outcome of these trials can be partly explained by poor long-term compliance to changes in diet, coupled with significant improvements in coronary health care [20], an over-emphasis on serum cholesterol as a therapeutic target is also likely to be involved.

The risk attributable to raised total serum and LDL cholesterol within populations (population-attributable risk) is actually lower than might be expected. The absolute risk associated with a serum cholesterol of 7.8 mmol/l is about 90%, as derived from epidemiological mortality curves. However, a considerable proportion of many populations (~50%) have serum cholesterol values between 5.2 and 6.5 mmol/l. In diagnostic terms this is often referred to as a 'grey area' since serum cholesterol in this range does not discriminate between individuals with coronary disease and those without [21, 22]. The population-attributable risk in this range is three-fold higher than at serum cholesterol above 7.8 mmol/l. In other words, three times as many people will be 'at risk' in this range but this risk in absolute terms is only about 20%. Another way to view this is through the disparity in the incidence of coronary heart disease amongst individuals with equivalent serum LDL cholesterol values, ie between 5.2–6.5 mmol/l. This can be explained by the existence of other risk factors, many of which may impinge on the risk associated with serum cholesterol and even modify the potential atherogenicity of cholesterol-carrying lipoproteins such as LDL. Serum triglycerides (TG) represent such a risk factor [23].

Moderately-raised serum TG (>1.5 mmol/l) can radically alter the physical form of LDL and HDL so that they become small and dense particles with aberrant metabolic qualities. This transformation dramatically increases the atherogenicity of LDL and decreases the capacity to transport cholesterol from tissues via HDL. Reductions in HDL can also impair the catabolism of TG-rich lipoproteins which exacerbates the raised serum TG still further. These changes are associated with a three- to four-fold increase in coronary risk [24] and may represent the most common source of lipid-mediated cardiovascular risk in free-living populations. Most importantly, raised serum TG is considerably more responsive than serum cholesterol to changes in lifestyle and diet. The concentration of serum cholesterol provides no information on the level of serum TG. Likewise, dietary cholesterol has no affect on serum TG or its associated abnormalities in LDL and HDL.

References

1 Weinhouse S. The blood cholesterol. Archs Path 1943:35, 438–500.
2 Stamler J, Wentworth D, Neaton JD. Is the relationship between serum cholesterol and risk of premature death from coronary heart disease continuous and graded? The Multiple Risk Factor Intervention Trial. JAMA 1986:256, 2823–8.
3 Smith EB, Slater RS. Relationship between low-density lipoprotein in aortic intima and serum-lipid levels. Lancet i, 1972: 463–9.
4 Scandinavian Simvastatin Survival Study Group. Randomized trial of cholesterol lowering in 4444 patients with coronary heart disease: the Scandanavian Simvastatin Survival Study (4S). Lancet 1994:344, 383–9.
5 Shepherd J, Cobbe SM, Ford I, Isles CG, Lorimer AR, MacFarlane PW, McKillop JH, Packard CJ. Prevention of coronary heart disease with pravastatin in men with hypercholesterolaemia: West of Scotland Coronary Prevention Study Group. New Eng J Med 1995:333, 1301–7.
6 Keys A. Coronary heart disease in seven countries. Circulation 1970: 41, Suppl. 1 I-186 to I-198.
7 Haq IU, Yeo WW, Jackson PR, Ramsay LE. The effects of dietary change on serum cholesterol. Proc Nutr Soc 1995:54, 601–16.
8 Brown MS, Faust JR, Goldstein JL. Role of the low density lipoprotein receptor in regulating the content of free and esterified cholesterol in human fibroblasts. J Clin Invest 1975:55, 783–93.
9 Anitshkow N. Changes in rabbit aorta due to experimentally induced cholesterolsteatosis. Beitr Path Anat Allegem Path 1913:56, 379–404.
10 Mistry P, Miller NE, Laker M, Hazzard WR, Lewis B. Individual variation in the effects of dietary cholesterol on plasma lipoproteins and cellular cholesterol homeostasis in man. J Clin Invest 1981:67, 493–502.
11 Packard CJ, McKinney L, Carr K, Shepherd J. Cholesterol feeding increases low density lipoprotein synthesis. J Clin Invest 1983:72, 45–51.
12 Committee on Medical Aspects of Food Policy (COMA). Nutritional aspects of cardiovascular disease. DH Rept Hlth Soc Subj 1994:46.

13 Committee on Medical Aspects of Food Policy (COMA). Dietary reference values for food energy and nutrients for the United Kingdom. DH Rept Hlth Soc Subj 1991:41.
14 Durrington PN. Diet. In: Hyperlipidaemia: diagnosis and management, 1995, 225–57. London: Butterworth-Heinemann.
15 Ostlund Jr RE, Bosner MS, Stenson WF. Cholesterol absorption efficiency declines at moderate dietary doses in normal human subjects. J Lip Res 1999:40, 1453–8.
16 Sehayek E, Nath C, Heinemann T, McGee M, Seiman CE, Samuel P, Breslow JL. U-shape relationship between change in dietary cholesterol absorption and plasma lipoprotein responsiveness and evidence for extreme interindividual variation in dietary cholesterol absorption in humans. J Lip Res 1998:39, 2415–22.
17 Wu LH, James T, Hopkins PN. Apolipoprotein E: Laboratory determinations and clinical significance. In: Handbook of lipoprotein testing (Rifai et al eds), 1997, pp329-356. American Association for Clinical Chemistry.
18 Kesaniemi YA, Ehnholm C, Miettinen TA. Intestinal cholesterol absorption efficiency in man is related to apoprotein E phenotype. J Clin Invest 1987:80, 578–81.
19 Glatz JFC, Demacker PNM, Turner PR, Katan MB. Response of serum cholesterol to dietary cholesterol in relation to apolipoprotein E phenotype. Nutr Metab Cardiovasc Dis 1991:1, 13–17.
20 Tunstall-Pedoe H, Vanuzzo D, Hobbs M, Mahonen M, Cepaitis Z, Kuulasmaa K, Keil U. Estimation of contribution of changes in coronary care to improving survival, event rates, and coronary heart disease mortality across the WHO MONICA Project populations. Lancet: 355, 668–9.
21 Castelli WP. Epidemiology of coronary heart disease: The Framingham study. Am J Med 1984: 76(2A), 4–12.
22 Fruchart JC, Packard CJ. Is cholesterol the major lipoprotein risk factor in coronary heart disease? – a Franco-Scottish overview. Cur Med Res Opinion 1997:13, 603–16.
23 Hokanson J, Austin MA. Plasma triglyceride level is a risk factor for cardio-vascular disease independent of high-density lipoprotein cholesterol: a meta-analysis of population-based prospective studies. J Cardiovasc Risk 1996:3, 213–19.
24 Griffin BA, Freeman DJ, Tait GW, Thomson J, Caslake MJ, Packard CJ, Shepherd J. Role of plasma triglyceride in the regulation of plasma low density lipoprotein (LDL) subfractions: relative contribution of small, dense LDL to coronary heart disease risk. Atherosclerosis 1994:106, 241–53.
25 Ginsberg HN, Karmally W, Siddiqui M, Holleran S, Tall AR, Rumsey et al. A dose-response study of the effects of dietary cholesterol on fasting and postprandial lipid and lipoprotein metabolism in healthy young men. Arterioscl Thromb 1994:14, 576–86.
26 Schnohr P, Thomsen OO, Hansen R, Boberg-Ans G, Lawaetz H, Weeke T. Egg consumption and high-density lipoprotein cholesterol. J Int Med 1994:235, 249–51.
27 Vuoristo M, Miettinen TA. Absorption, metabolism and serum concentrations of cholesterol in vegetarians: effects of cholesterol feeding. Am J Clin Nutr 1994:59, 1325–31.
28 Kern Jr F. Effects of dietary cholesterol on cholesterol and bile acid homeostasis in patients with cholesterol gallstones. J Clin Invest 1994:93, 1186–94.
29 Ginsberg HN, Karmally W, Siddiqui M, Holleran S. Increases in dietary cholesterol are associated with modest increases in both LDL and HDL cholesterol in healthy young women. Arterioscl Thromb Vasc Biol 1995:15, 169–78.
30 Knopp H. A double-blind, randomized trial of the effects of two eggs per day in moderately hypercholesterolemic and combined hyperlipidemic subjects consuming the NCEP Step I diet. American Heart Association, Anaheim, CA. 1995.
31 Clifton PM, Noakes M, Nestel PI. LDL particle size and LDL and HDL cholesterol changes with dietary fat and cholesterol in healthy subjects. J Lipid Res 1998:39, 1799–804.

Dietary cholesterol as a cardiac risk factor: myth or reality? Ed Anthony R Leeds, Juliet Gray. ©2001. Smith-Gordon. Printed in UK.

3 *Genetic influence on cholesterol absorption and its therapeutic consequences*

Gilbert R. Thompson

Emeritus Professor of Clinical Lipidology, Imperial College, London, UK.

Wide variations in the response of serum cholesterol to changes in the amount of cholesterol in the diet are well documented in both animals and man. Genetic factors which regulate cholesterol absorption almost certainly play a major role in determining interindividual variability of response to changes in intake. However, the precise mechanism whereby cholesterol is selectively transported into the enterocyte remains uncertain. Recent data suggest that an important determinant of net absorption of cholesterol is the amount which effluxes back into the intestinal lumen, a process which is regulated by the ATP-binding cassette transporter 1 (ABC 1). Genetic variation at this key regulatory step could be responsible at least in part for hypo- and hyper-responsiveness to dietary cholesterol.

Another probable genetic influence is possession of an apoE4 allele, which predisposes to hyper-responsiveness to dietary cholesterol but hypo-responsiveness to statin therapy. Poor responders to statins are characterised by high absorption but low synthesis of cholesterol. Concomitant ingestion of plant stanol esters, which block cholesterol absorption and thereby upregulate endogenous synthesis, might help improve the response of individuals who are refractory to statin therapy.

Animal studies

The effect of a 0.5% cholesterol diet on the serum cholesterol of six in-bred strains of rabbits was examined by Beynen et al [1], as shown in Fig. 1. Their cholesterol levels on a normal rabbit chow diet, shown by the black histograms, were all similarly low but each strain, when put on the high cholesterol diet, responded differently with increases in serum cholesterol which ranged from less than 10 mmol/l to up to 40 mmol/l.

The mechanism which might determine hypo- and hyper-responsiveness to dietary cholesterol was explored recently by Dietschy and colleagues [2] using two strains of mice called C57 Black/6 and 129/Sv. Irrespective of whether they were on a diet containing no added cholesterol, added cholesterol, cholesterol plus saturated fat or cholesterol plus monounsaturated fat, the Black 6 strain always showed a less marked increase in plasma cholesterol than the 129/Sv strain. This difference not only applied to plasma cholesterol but also to the concentration of cholesterol in the livers of these animals. To investigate the possible basis for the difference between the response of the two strains, the Dallas group first measured total lipid absorption and found that each strain was equally good at absorbing dietary fat which, of

---

Address for correspondence: Professor G.R. Thompson, Metabolic Medicine, Imperial College School of Medicine, Hammersmith Hospital, London W12 0NN, UK.

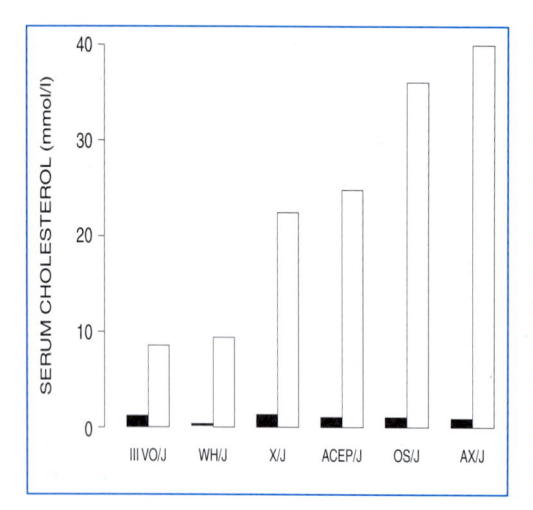

Figure 1. Effect of 0.5% cholesterol diet on serum cholesterol in six inbred strains of rabbits (reproduced with permission from Beynen et al [1]).

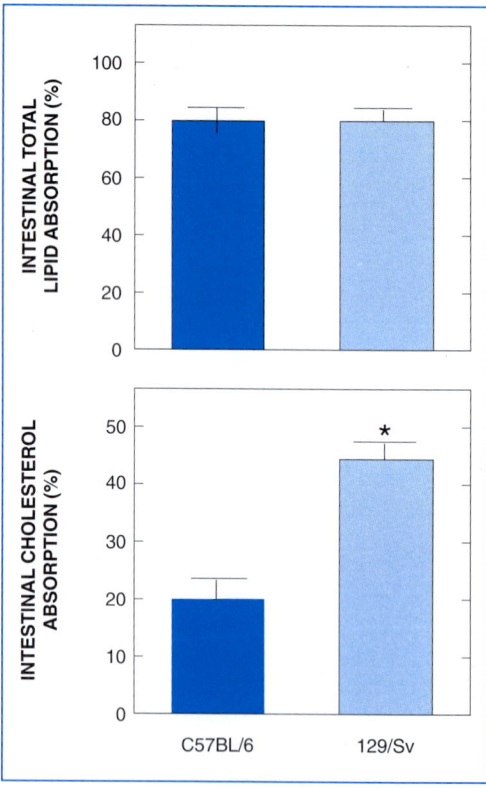

Figure 2. Total lipid and cholesterol absorption in C57BL/6 and 129/Sv strains of mice (reproduced with permission from Jolley et al [2]).

course, is mainly triglyceride (Fig. 2, upper panel). However, when they examined intestinal cholesterol absorption, the hypo-responsive strain absorbed less than half as much dietary cholesterol as the hyper-responsive strain (Fig. 2, lower panel). This suggests that at least one reason for hypo- or hyper-responsiveness is the efficiency with which dietary cholesterol is absorbed. In contrast, rates of cholesterol synthesis in both the liver and the small intestine were much higher in the hypo-responders than in the hyper-responders. Thus, it seems as if it is the amount of cholesterol that is absorbed from the diet, at least in mice, rather than the rate of endogenous cholesterol synthesis, which determines diet-induced changes in blood cholesterol.

Human studies

If we now turn to man, Mistry et al [3] fed six egg yolks a day for 2 weeks to 37 normal subjects and showed quite marked differences in response between individuals. The mean change in serum cholesterol was a rise of 0.75 mmol/l, most of the people in this study showing a rise in serum cholesterol which ranged from 0.1 to 1.9 mmol/l. A minority showed either no change or a small decrease (–0.16 mmol/l). This was a short-term study, rather artificial in that few people eat six eggs a week, let alone six a day, but it does illustrate that inter-individual differences in response to dietary cholesterol exist in man as in animals.

These differences in response are reproducible to some extent in that hypo-responders whose cholesterol intake is raised from the region of 120–130 to 625–990 mg per day always seem to show a less marked increase in serum cholesterol than do hyper-responders, even though the changes within each group are not particularly consistent [1]. These findings suggest the existence of a genetic basis for inter-individual differences in responsiveness to dietary cholesterol in man, as in mice.

Mechanistic studies

To investigate the reasons for this phenome-

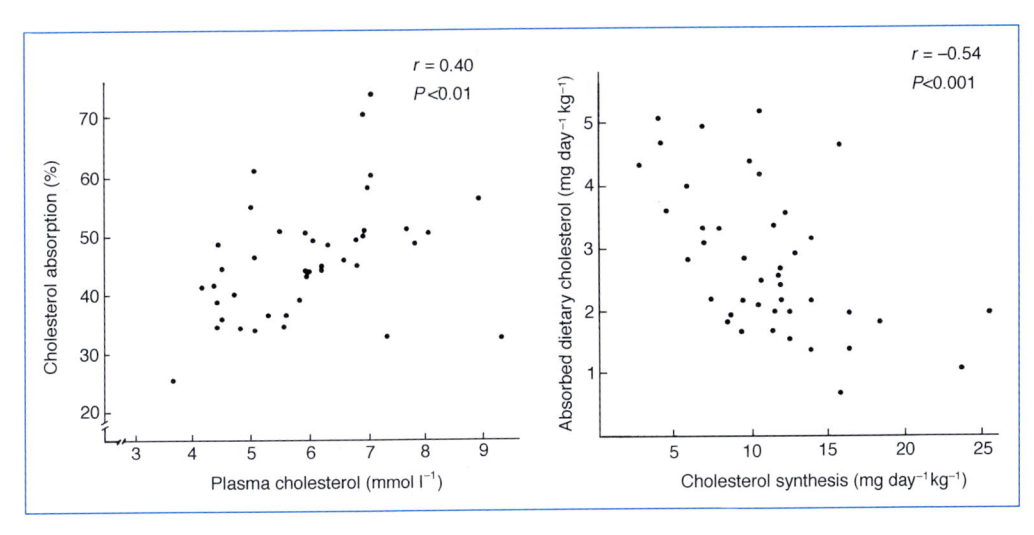

Figure 3. Correlations between (left) plasma cholesterol and percent cholesterol absorption and (right) between cholesterol absorption and synthesis (reproduced with permission from Kesaniemi and Miettinen [4]).

non, Kataan and colleagues measured increases in serum cholesterol on low and on high cholesterol intakes and correlated the changes with whole-body cholesterol synthesis [1]. The people who showed the greatest increase in serum cholesterol on a high cholesterol intake had the lowest basal rate of cholesterol synthesis before being put onto the high cholesterol diet, whereas the people who showed only small increases had higher basal rates of cholesterol synthesis. These findings are similar to those in mice where the Black 6 strain had a higher rate of cholesterol synthesis than the 1 29/Sv strain and a less marked increase in plasma cholesterol when they were put on a high cholesterol intake [2].

Another study, from Finland, examined not only the relationship between plasma cholesterol and cholesterol synthesis, but also cholesterol absorption [4]. As shown in Fig. 3, people whose plasma cholesterol on their normal diet is in the high range, tend to be more efficient absorbers of cholesterol in percentage terms than those whose plasma cholesterol is at the low or normal end of the range. Hence, people with a high serum cholesterol, and those who show an exaggerated response to dietary cholesterol, tend to hyper-absorb dietary cholesterol and have a low rate of cholesterol synthesis, whereas people who absorb the least have a lower serum cholesterol despite a higher rate of synthesis.

Candidate genes regulating cholesterol absorption

Which genes might be responsible for determining differences in the ability to absorb cholesterol? Among those which have been suggested are caveolin, the scavenger receptor class B type 1, sterol carrier protein and intestinal acyl cholesterol acyl transferase (ACAT), which is involved in the re-esterification of cholesterol after it has crossed the brush border of the intestinal mucosa [2]. However, these suggestions are largely hypothetical with little in the way of hard evidence to support them. Two more likely candidate genes are those specifying apoE phenotype and the ATP binding cassette transporter protein, known as ABC 1. The latter mediates the efflux of cholesterol from peripheral tissues and is the source of the cholesterol which leads to the formation of HDL. In patients with Tangier disease, who have mutations of this gene, there is no efflux; this results in accumulation of cholesterol in tissues, particularly in the tonsils, and the virtual absence of HDL from plasma.

Normally, mice respond to increases in

dietary cholesterol by reducing the efficiency of absorption [5]. This is a well-recognised phenomenon which not only occurs in mice but also in man. Ostlund et al [6] used a stable isotopic method to measure cholesterol absorption in two groups of subjects, each of whom were studied on a low intake of cholesterol (26 mg) and then on a higher intake, either 188 mg or 421 mg daily. The percentage absorption of cholesterol was lower on the higher intake in both groups, especially in those fed more than 400 mg a day. Within both these groups, some people responded with a dramatic reduction in cholesterol absorption on the higher dose whereas in others cholesterol absorption hardly changed.

Recently, McNeish et al [7] reported the results of studies carried out in ABC1 knock-out mice while on a low-cholesterol chow diet and also while on a high cholesterol diet. As shown in Table 1, in normal intact mice (ABC1 +/+) the efficiency of absorption decreased from 69 to 49% when they were fed a high cholesterol diet. In contrast, the ABC1 gene knock-out mice (ABC1 –/–) absorb cholesterol more efficiently than normal mice on the chow diet and continue to absorb it efficiently even when they are given the high cholesterol diet. Now, as stated earlier, the function of ABC1 is to promote the efflux of cholesterol from cells and the implication of these results is that if you knock out the gene for this transporter, intestinal efflux of cholesterol is blocked. In normal mice, when they are fed the high cholesterol diet, the amount of cholesterol re-excreted into the intestine is increased by up-regulation of ABC1 and net absorption decreases. If ABC1 has been knocked out, cholesterol is solely transported inwards and there is no efflux to balance any increase in cholesterol intake. Thus genetic polymorphism of ABC1 could explain variations in response to dietary cholesterol.

Which brings us to apoE. Very similar studies have been carried out in mice who have an intact apoE gene or in whom the latter had been knocked out [8]. When they were switched from a low to a high cholesterol intake, the apoE intact mice responded like the ABC1 intact mice by decreasing their absorption of cholesterol. However, the apoE knock-out mice were unable to adapt and continued to absorb cholesterol efficiently and became very hypercholesterolaemic.

The existence of apoE polymorphism in humans has been alluded to already and the three major alleles have been described. The normal apoE genotype, 3/3, is possessed by two-thirds of the population, whereas about 20% have the E3/4 genotype. A small minority, probably less than 5% have the E4/4 genotype, except in Finland where there is a very high prevalence of the E4 allele. Sarkinnen et al [9] examined the effect of an NCEP step 1 diet without and with the addition of 300 mg of cholesterol on the serum cholesterol of three groups of Finns according to their apoE genotype. As shown in Fig. 4, they remained on their baseline diet for the first 4 weeks and were then placed on a NCEP step 1 diet. All three groups showed a decrease in serum cholesterol by 6 weeks. They remained on this diet for 12 weeks at the end of which the great-

Table 1 Cholesterol absorption in ABC1 knock-out mice (McNeish et al [7]).

Diet	ABC1 +/+	ABC1 –/–
Chow	69 ± 6%	81 ± 9%*
High cholesterol	49 ± 11%	79 ± 8%**

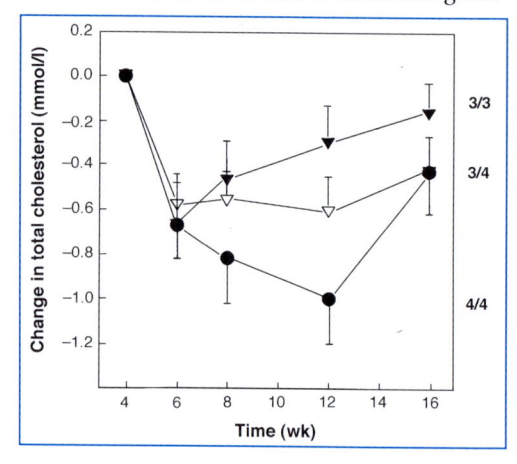

* = P<0.05   ** = P<0.005

Figure 4. Effect of NCEP step 1 diet without and with addition of cholesterol 300 mg/day on serum cholesterol according to apoE genotype. Weeks: 0–4, baseline diet; 4–12, step 1; 12–16, step 1 + egg yolks. (Adapted with permission from Sarkinnen et al [9].)

est fall was in the E4/4s, the least in the 3/3s, with the 3/4s intermediate. They then continued with their step 1 diet, but with the addition of 300 mg of cholesterol daily. The subsequent rise in cholesterol in the E4/4s was greater than in 3/4s and 3/3s. This suggests that individuals homozygous for E4 show exaggerated responses to removal of cholesterol and saturated fat from the diet, as well as to the addition of cholesterol without any change in the fat content of the diet, as compared with people with a normal apoE phenotype.

Another Finnish study showed that people who have an E4 allele are more efficient at absorbing cholesterol and had lower synthetic rates than those with the normal phenotype [10]. Hence, those with an E4 allele, who are often hypercholesterolaemic to start with and show an exaggerated response to dietary cholesterol, tend to be efficient absorbers and low synthesisers of cholesterol.

Clinical consequences

What are the clinical implications of these putative genetic influences? Most people are familiar with the Scandinavian Simvastatin Survival Study, 4S, which changed the practice of medicine throughout the whole world and especially the management of coronary disease. One of the many sub-group analyses conducted on the results of 4S was by Miettinen et al [11] and involved the Finnish cohort, who numbered in the region of 800 people. These were divided into quartiles according to their cholestanol to cholesterol ratio. Cholestanol was used as an index of cholesterol absorption and correlates very closely with the serum level of campesterol, another marker of cholesterol absorption. As shown in Fig. 5, those in the lowest quartile of the cholestanol to cholesterol ratio were regarded as hypo-absorbers, those in the highest quartile as hyper-absorbers. As in previous studies, an inverse correlation between cholesterol absorption and synthesis is evident, synthesis here being indicated by the ratio of lathosterol to cholesterol; thus people who absorb less cholesterol, synthesise more and vice versa.

When the changes in serum cholesterol in the Finnish sub-group on placebo were examined according to cholestanol to cholesterol ratios, there were no differences between the people in the lowest quartile, Q1, and those in the highest quartile, Q4. However, when the sub-group who were treated with simvastatin were examined, it was found that the reduction in serum cholesterol in Q4, the people who absorbed a lot of cholesterol and synthesised a little, was less marked than in Q1, the people who absorbed less and synthesised more. The probable reason for this difference was that the people in the fourth quartile showed a less marked decrease in their lathosterol:cholesterol ratio (Fig. 5) when on simvastatin, the action of which is to inhibit cholesterol synthesis, than the people in the first quartile. In other words, people whose synthesis rate is low to start with, show a lesser decrease in synthesis when they are treated with simvastatin than those people whose synthesis rate is initially high.

Miettinen et al [12] also looked at the reduction in risk of coronary events in 4S according to the quartiles of the cholestanol to cholesterol ratio. As shown in Table 2, the ratios in these quartiles ranged from less than 107 to

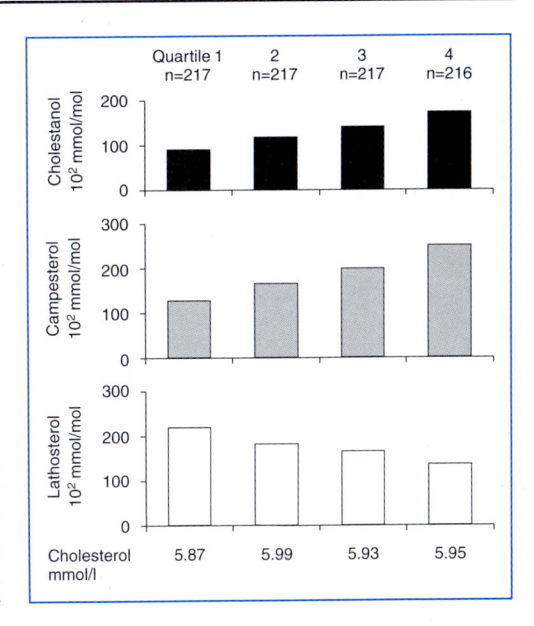

Figure 5. Baseline ratios of markers of cholesterol absorption and synthesis according to quartiles of the cholestanol:cholesterol ratio in plasma of Finnish cohort of 4S (based on data from Miettinen et al [1]).

Table 2 Reduction in risk of CHD events by simvastatin according to baseline cholestanol (Miettinen et al [12]).

	Quartiles			
	1st	2nd	3rd	4th
Cholestanol:cholesterol*	<107	107–126	127–148	>148
Relative risk of CHD	0.62‡	0.66	0.75	1.17‡

* 10^2 mmol/mol ‡$P<0.01$

more than 148, expressed as 10^2 mmol of cholestanol per mol of cholesterol. The relative risk of coronary heart disease in simvastatin-treated subjects in the first and second quartiles was reduced by 34–38% and by 25% in the third quartile, but it was not reduced, in fact if anything the risk was increased, in those in the fourth quartile. In other words, people who had a high cholestanol to cholesterol ratio at the start of the trial, that is to say the high absorbers and low synthesisers, did not show any reduction in coronary events when they were treated with simvastatin and in fact had the same relative risk as placebo-treated subjects.

Using mevalonic acid rather than lathosterol as an index of cholesterol synthesis, Naoumova et al [13] also found that a poor response to statins was associated with a low basal rate of cholesterol synthesis. The possibility that this phenomenon may sometimes be due to inheritance of the apoE4 allele has been documented by Ordovas et al [14], presumably via the associated increase in cholesterol absorption.

Therapeutic implications

What can be done to improve the outcome of people who respond poorly to statins? One possible approach is to try to inhibit their absorption of cholesterol, which of course includes not just dietary cholesterol but also the endogenous cholesterol entering the intestine via the bile duct. It is well established that margarines like Benecol, which contain plant stanol esters, block the absorption of cholesterol from the intestine and upregulate cholesterol synthesis. The published results of randomised, placebo-controlled studies of at least 3 weeks' duration show that plant stanol esters exert a dose-dependent effect on LDL cholesterol, reductions ranging from 10% with 1–2 g stanol/day to 13% with 2–3 g/day.

Hence, one way of possibly making subjects known to be unresponsive to statins more responsive is to block their cholesterol absorption by giving them plant stanol or sterol esters and upregulating their HMG CoA reductase. There have already been a couple of studies suggesting that the combination of stanols and statins is a good one and that they are additive in their effects on LDL [15, 16]. However, it remains to be shown whether the response of poor responders is increased to an even greater extent than that of good responders by this approach.

References

1 Beynen AC, Katan MB, Van Zutphen LF. Hypo- and hyperresponders: individual differences in the response of serum cholesterol concentration to changes in diet. Adv Lipid Res 1987:22, 115–71.
2 Jolley CD, Dietschy JM, Turley SD. Genetic differences in cholesterol absorption in 129/Sv and C57BL/6 mice: effect on cholesterol responsiveness. Am J Physiol 1999:276, G1117–24.
3 Mistry P, Miller NE, Laker M, Hazzard WR, Lewis B. Individual variation in the effects of dietary cholesterol on plasma lipoproteins and cellular cholesterol homeostasis in man. Studies of low density lipoprotein receptor activity and 3-hydroxy-3-methylglutaryl coenzyme A reductase activity in blood mononuclear cells. J Clin Invest 1981:67, 493–502.
4 Kesaniemi YA, Miettinen TA. Cholesterol absorption efficiency regulates plasma cholesterol level in the Finnish population. Eur J Clin Invest 1987:17, 391–5.
5 Sehayek E, Ono JG, Shefer S, Nguyen LB, Wang N, Batta AK, Salen G, Smith JD, Tall AR, Breslow JL. Biliary cholesterol excretion: a novel mechanism that regulates cholesterol absorption. Proc Natl Acad Sci USA 1998:95, 10194–9.
6 Ostlung RE Jr, Bosner MS, Stenson WF. Cholesterol absorption efficiency declines at moderate dietary doses in normal human subjects. J Lipid Res 1999:40, 1453–8.
7 McNeish J, Aiello RJ, Guyot D, Turi T, Gabel C, Aldinger C, Hoppe KL, Roach ML, Royer U, de Wet J, Broccardo C, Chimini G, Francone OL. High density lipoprotein deficiency and foam

8. Sehayek E, Shefer S, Nguyen LB, Ono JG, Merkel M, Breslow JL. Apolipoprotein E regulates dietary cholesterol absorption and biliary cholesterol excretion: studies in C57BL/6 apolipoprotein E knockout mice. Proc Natl Acad Sci USA 2000:97, 3433–7.

cell accumulation in mice with targeted disruption of ATP-binding cassette transporter-1. Proc Natl Acad Sci USA 2000:97, 4245–50.

9. Sarkkinen E, Korhonen M, Erkkila A, Ebeling T, Uusitupa M. Effect of apolipoprotein E polymorphism on serum lipid response to the separate modification of dietary fat and dietary cholesterol. Am J Clin Nutr 1998:68, 1215–22.

10. Kesaniemi YA, Enholm C, Miettinen TA. Intestinal cholesterol absorption efficiency in man is related to apoprotein E phenotype. J Clin Invest 1987:80, 578–81.

11. Miettinen TA, Strandberg TE, Gylling H, for the Finnish Investigators of the Scandinavian Simvastatin Survival Study Group. Noncholesterol sterols and cholesterol lowering by long-term simvastatin treatment in coronary patients. Relation to basal serum cholesterol. Arterioscler Thromb Vasc Biol 2000:20, 1340–46.

12. Miettinen TA, Gylling H, Strandberg T, Sarna S, for the Finnish 4S Investigators. Baseline serum cholestanol as predictor of recurrent coronary events in subgroup of Scandinavian Simvastatin Survival Study. Br Med J 1998:316, 1127–30.

13. Naoumova RP, Marais AD, Mountney J, Firth JC, Rendell NB, Taylor GW, Thompson GR. Plasma mevalonic acid, an index of cholesterol synthesis in vivo, and responsiveness to HMG CoA reductase inhibitors in familial hypercholeterolaemia. Atherosclerosis 1996:119, 203–13.

14. Ordovas JM, Lopez-Miranda J, Perez-Jimenez F, Rodriguez C, Park J-S, Cole T, Schaefer EJ. Effect of apolipoprotein E and A-IV phenotypes on the low density lipoprotein response to HMG CoA reductase inhibitor therapy. Atherosclerosis 1995:113, 157–66.

15. Vuorio AF, Gylling H, Turtola H, Kontula K, Ketonen P, Miettinen TA. Stanol ester margarine alone and with simvastatin lowers serum cholesterol in families with familial hypercholesterolaemia caused by the FH–North Karelia mutation. Arterioscler Thromb Vasc Biol 2000:20, 500–6.

16. Blair SN, Capuzzi DM, Gottlieb SO, Nguyen T, Morgan JM, Cater NB. Incremental reduction of serum total cholesterol and low-density lipoprotein cholesterol with the addition of plant stanol ester-containing spread to statin therapy. Am J Cardiol 2000:86, 46–52.

Dietary cholesterol as a cardiac risk factor: myth or reality? Ed Anthony R Leeds, Juliet Gray. ©2001. Smith-Gordon. Printed in UK.

4   *Dietary cholesterol as a cardiac risk factor: current dietetic practice*

Gary Frost

Department of Nutrition and Dietetics, Hammersmith Hospital, London, UK.

The overview of the significance of dietary cholesterol is that in amounts normally eaten in the diet it has very little effect on coronary heart disease risk. There are many dietary risk factors that play an important role in reducing cardiac risk. The success of lifestyle advice could be maximised through simple measures such as consistent messages.

Introduction

Focusing on one aspect of dietary management of coronary artery disease, in this case dietary cholesterol, simplifies what is not a simple problem. This has been nicely demonstrated recently with the update to Ashwell's round table of cardiac risk [1], see Fig. 1.

This demonstrates the complex interplay between risk factors and the need for equal consideration to be given to diet, exercise, body weight, and pharmacological intervention in managing these risk factors. For this reason in this chapter I would like to broaden the topic to include a discussion of dietary risk management of a broad base of coronary-heart-disease risk factors. In clinical practice it is relatively rare to have a patient being treated with one cardiac risk factor. Usually patients have a complex web of both modifiable (serum cholesterol, hypertension, diabetes, obesity) and non-modifiable risk factors (age, sex, family history). It is the assessment of all of these risk factors that will dictate the type of therapy and the way it is applied. So the purpose of this chapter is to present an overview of dietary risk management.

Good team-work, with good internal communications between team members, is very important if the effects of lifestyle advice are to be maximised. Conflicting messages about treatment undermine the effectiveness of the therapy. It is essential that the team members, be it a lipid team or GP practice, all know the aims of what they are trying to achieve with a patient and how these will be achieved. One of the main issues with nutritional advice is consistency of message. If one member of the team says weight is the main focus, and another says weight is not important but changing to polyunsaturated fat is, clearly this creates confusion for the patient and undermines the patient's faith in health professionals knowing what they are taking about. Within the team there needs to be an agreed method of tackling coronary risk factors. Perhaps one way is the adoption of risk factor management tables and treatment pathways.

Auditing the effectiveness of advice on lipid-lowering to patients should reflect the approach of the team as a whole rather than an individual health-care professional.

This chapter will first consider the science

Address for correspondence: Dr Gary Frost, Head of Nutrition and Dietetic Research Group, Department of Nutrition and Dietetics, Hammersmith Hospital, DuCane Road, London W12 0HS, UK.

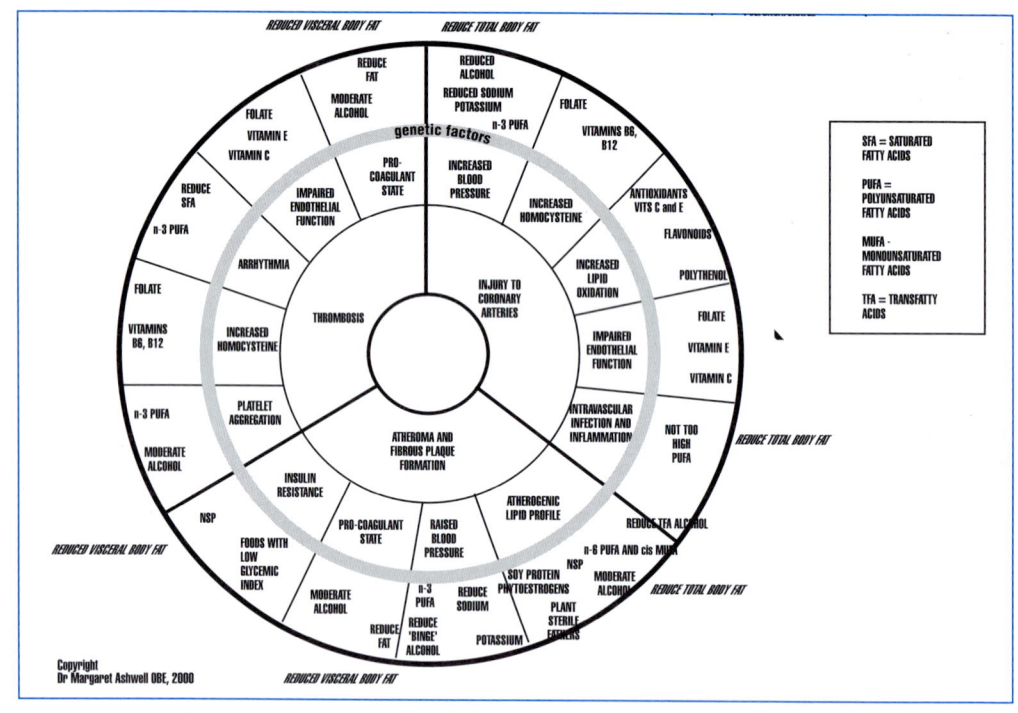

Figure 1. A round table of dietary and other factors in the prevention of coronary heart disease [1].

behind modern-day advice for cardiac risk factor reduction before, secondly, suggesting how the science may be put into practice and the health message made clearer to the patient.

Science behind the advice

Complex interplay

The complex interplay between risk factors is exemplified by the insulin resistance syndrome [2]. The syndrome is exemplified by hyperinsulinaemia and the related risk factors of abnormal glucose metabolism, hypertriglycaemia, low high-density lipoprotein cholesterol, abnormal post-prandial lipaemia, hypertension and abnormal clotting factors. It is unlikely that a single lifestyle intervention will have an effect on all of these risk factors. The challenge for the future is to try and reflect this multiple risk factor picture into advice that has been demonstrated to improve syndromes such as insulin resistance.

Dietary cholesterol

This has been covered in the chapters that precede this one. Basically the intervention studies that demonstrate that dietary cholesterol has a detrimental effect on serum cholesterol have used amounts of dietary cholesterol that are in excess of normal intake [3]. Classic studies that have looked at the effect of cholesterol in the 'normal' diet have failed to show any effect [4]. There is variation in physiological response which possibly relates to genetic susceptibility [5]. Overall the message seems to be that the intake of dietary cholesterol within a physiological range has little impact on serum cholesterol levels or coronary heart disease risk. This is important as clinical practice is concerned with the risk of a dietary component eaten in amounts that can be consumed in the diet not in pharmacological dosages.

Obesity management

There continues to be an exponential increase in the percentage of the population who are overweight or obese. Current estimates for the UK population are that 50–60% are overweight and nearly 20% are obese [6]. The relationship between obesity and a number of cardiac risk factors, such as total cholesterol, low HDL-cholesterol, high TG, hyperinsulinaemia, abnormal clotting profiles, is irrefutable. More recently the academic argument over whether obesity is an independent risk factor has received positive support for the proposition with the publication of work from the Nurses' Health Study [7]. A large proportion of people presenting with multiple cardiac risk factors are obese or overweight. A major at-risk population is type-2 diabetic patients; in this group 80% are overweight. Effective management of obesity can have dramatic effects on all cardiac risk factors.

It is only recently that we have started to get to grips with understanding the importance of weight management. It is a new era and I feel that we are moving towards a time of effective management of obesity. A few years ago it could have been argued that treatment was not very effective. There is a new age now which possibly started in the UK with the publication of the Scottish SIGN document [8] on the management of obesity. This has been followed-up with the publication of the Royal College of Physicians of England, which had a similar approach. These reports highlighted the effectiveness of a small amount of weight loss on mortality and cardiac risk factors. In those with one or more risk factors for CHD, or who have established CHD, a weight loss of as little as 5% can produce marked changes in risk profile. In those without obvious risk factors 10% weight loss has been shown to have marked effects.

As far as dietary management of obesity is concerned, the understanding of how small amounts of weight loss have dramatic effects on cardiac risk factors means there has been a move away from unachievable targets of 'normal body weight'.

Another influence on management is the understanding that large energy deficits are unsustainable and therefore fail. Small energy deficits of <500 kcal, although they produce slow initial weight loss, are more sustainable over time and produce greater weight loss [9]. These reports highlight the importance of having treatment pathways that will cover health education through primary care to surgical intervention in order to offer a co-ordinated service to the obese. Before embarking on a weight-loss programme there is a need to find answers to some questions:

- Does the patient sign-up to weight loss?
- Do the patients want to change their diet?

These are fundamental parts of the 'helping people change' model of care, without the answers to these questions it is impossible to move forward [10].

It is up to dietitians as a profession to embrace these concepts and accept that, as with functional foods, and food-based guidelines, if management is to be effective we need many tools to help. These may range from very-low-calorie diets to drug therapy to surgical intervention. Ongoing studies such as the Swedish Obesity Study may help inform practice [11]. More locally, initiatives such as the Counterweight programme may help inform pratice in primary care [12].

Fat and fatty acids

Keys's classic studies and others since then have demonstrated the direct relationship between dietary fat intake and plasma cholesterol levels [3]. They have been backed up by randomised control trials that demonstrate that when total fat intake is increased total cholesterol and LDL cholesterol increase and HDL decreases. However, this picture has become complicated by increasing knowledge of the properties of many individual fatty acids. In the future we may see a movement towards advice on individual fatty acids. In practice there is very little thought given to this. Rarely is it considered that stearic acid consumption is associated with lower LDL-cholesterol. Even fish oils, which have a demonstrated track record in reducing secondary events, as shown by the DART study [13], are often ignored in favour of a general focus on fats.

Functional foods

Functional foods, such as those that have been enriched with the likes of plant stanols/sterols, and which come with a first-class research background, need to be embraced. There have been randomised control trials that demonstrate a 15–20% reduction in total cholesterol, which has enormous potential benefits to public health problems [14]. There are problems with the cost of these products, which will make them basically unaffordable for those on a limited budget. This may change when there is competition from more than one product. Also energy intake needs to be considered in the obese when advising on a clinically relevant intake.

There is much excitement about soya-based products, and their relationship to the reduction in cardiac risk factors, as well as about polyphenols from tea. These need to be investigated, and if shown to be effective and safe as all the evidence suggests, their use will need to be considered.

The dietetic profession needs to be able to respond and advise people on moving science into practice. Although encouraging change in eating habits, along the lines of healthy eating guidelines, will remain the backbone of dietary advice for people at risk of CHD we must not get caught up in believing that the only way forward is through existing food-based guidelines. We need to be able to advise people on products which have been shown to have a positive benefit on health and are safe. This also enhances advice in the form that there is positive encouragement to eat something.

Limits to dietary advice

It is important to recognise the limits of dietary advice. Meta-analysis of cholesterol-lowering studies that were carried out under metabolic ward conditions demonstrated a reduction in blood cholesterol of 10–15% [15]. However, meta-analysis of studies in free-living populations showed a drop of 5% in total blood cholesterol [16]. The next section suggests a reason for this disparity. In exceptional circumstances large changes that affect vascular pathology can be achieved by lifestyle advice [17].

Getting the message across

The dietary approach has been the Cinderella of the management of cardiac risk factors and of many other diseases that require dietary intervention. We now have evidence from a variety of studies sufficient to suggest which dietary modification would be effective for an individual, for example low fat, low energy (weight loss), or modified carbohydrate. What we are not good at is convincing people to change their lifestyle. Very few counselling or education models have been subject to a randomised control trial. So at present the efficacy of advice is limited by the compliance of the individual. It has to be remembered that even in a meta-analysis of studies following dietary intervention the average 5% reduction in cholesterol recorded left 50% of the survey population who did not achieve that level [18].

There is urgent need for behaviour modification models that stand up to randomised control trials. There are a lot of simple questions, for example, are single messages better than multiple messages? This evidence is starting to trickle through. A recent paper by Steptoe et al [19] looked at change in cardiac risk factors in a randomised control trial of GP practices. In the intervention group the practice nurses were taught to counsel through helping people to change. Although there are problems with the study its experimental design is very robust [20]. It demonstrates that it is possible to run randomised trials on counselling models. There are a number of very simple areas that could make differences if they were demonstrated to make significant changes to lipid levels, for example:

- Does single message advice work?
- How effective is counselling to help people to change?

References

1 Ashwell MA, Hardman A, Oliver M. Cardiovascular disease risk: a round table approach. How do the factors related to diet, obesity, activity and drugs contribute to a combined strategy for prevention? Proc Nutr Soc 2000:59, 415–6.
2 Reavan GM. Syndrome X: 6 years later. J Intern Med 1994:236 (Supplement 736), 13–22.
3 Keys A, Anderson JT, Grande F. Serum cholestrol response to changes in diet. IV. Particularly saturated fatty acids in the diet. Metab Clin Exptl 1965:14, 776-87.
4 McNamara DJ. The impact of egg limitations on coronary heart disease risk: do the numbers add up? J Am Coll Nutr 2000:19, 540S–8S.
5 Williams R, Bhopal R, Hunt K. Coronary risk in a British Punjabi population: comparative profile

of non-biochemical factors. Int J Epidemiol 1994:23, 28–37.
6. Gregory J, Foster K, Tyler H, Wisemen M. The dietary and nutritional survey of British adults. Office of Population Censuses and Surveys. 1998. London, HMSO.
7. Houston MC. Hypertension and coronary heart disease risk factor management. Clin Auton Res 1993:3, 357–61.
8. Scottish Intercollegiate Guidelines Network (SIGN). Obesity in Scotland. Integrating prevention with weight management. 1999. Edinburgh, Royal College of Physicians.
9. Frost GS, Masters K, King C, Kelly M, Hasan U, Heavens P et al. A new method of energy prescription to improve weight loss. J Hum Nutr Diet 1991:4, 369–73.
10. Ni Mhurchu C, Margetts BM, Speller VM. Applying the stages-of-change model to dietary change. Nutr Rev 1997:55, 10–16.
11. Lissner L, Lindroos AK, Sjostrom L. Swedish obese subjects (SOS): an obesity intervention study with a nutritional perspective. Eur J Clin 1998: 52, 316–22.
12. Counterweight project board. The counterweight programme. European Study for Obesity (2000). Int J Obes. In press.
13. Burr ML, Gilbert JF, Holliday RM, Elwood PC, Fehily AM, Rogers S et al. Effects of changes in fat, fish, and fibre intakes on death and myocardial reinfarction: Diet and reinfarction trial (DART). Lancet 1989: 757–61.
14. Plat J, Kerckhoffs DAJM, Mensink RP. Therapeutic potential of plant sterols and stanols. Curr Opinion Lipidol 2000: 11, 571–6.
15. Clarke R, Frost C, Collins R, Appleby P, Peto R. Dietary lipids and blood cholesterol: a quantitative meta-analysis of metabolic ward studies. BMJ 1997:314, 112–17.
16. Tang JL, Armitage JM, Lancaster T, Silagy CA, Fowler GH, Neil HAW. Systematic review of dietary intervention trials to lower blood total cholesterol in free-living subjects. BMJ 1998:316, 1213–20.
17. Dunn G. Comparison of lifestyle and structured interventions to increase physical activity and cardiorespiratory fitness. JAMA 1999:281, 327–34.
18. Yu PS, Zhao GX, Etherton T, Naglak M, Jonnalagadda S, Kris-Etherton PM. Effects of the national cholesterol education program's step I and step II dietary intervention programs on cardiovascular disease risk factors: a meta-analysis. Am J Clin Nutr 1999:69(4), 632–46.
19. Steptoe A, Doherty S, Rink E, Kerry S, Kendrick T, Hilton S. Behavioural counselling in general practice for the promotion of healthy behaviour among adults at increased risk of coronary heart disease: randomised trial. BMJ 1999:319, 943–8.
20. Dore CJ, Frost G. Behavioural counselling in general practice about risk of CHD. Study had several methodological flaws. BMJ 2000:321, 49–50.

Dietary cholesterol as a cardiac risk factor: myth or reality? Ed Anthony R Leeds, Juliet Gray. ©2001. Smith-Gordon. Printed in UK.

5 Management of hypercholesterolaemia in primary health care – science into practice

John Ferguson

Prescription Pricing Authority (National Health Service), Newcastle Upon Tyne, UK.

The Medical Director of the Prescription Pricing Authority presents data on a number of key aspects of primary care approaches to hypercholesterolaemia. How did lipid-lowering drug usage develop in England in the 1990s? More recently what has been the pattern of statin prescribing? How much variation was there in the spending of 100 English Health Authorities? Was spending correlated with death rates? Do patterns of prescribing appear to be becoming more rational and potentially more effective? Against the picture that can be formed from such data there can be a debate about the best way to confront ischaemic heart disease in primary practice. Such a debate includes the role of cholesterol levels as a target of health prevention.

Personal background to practice in the last 10 years

As a medical student I remember an extremely dull series of biochemistry lectures. I thought that they were given by an extremely dull biochemist. However, I do remember what he had to say about cholesterol metabolism and that he explained in great detail the fact that it was a homeostatic mechanism. So as a result, I learnt that the amount the liver produced was related to the amount being taken in and absorbed. That, of course, explains why the dietary effects are as small as other speakers have already described today. This was in the pre-Keys 1965 days, so my 'dull' lecturer must have been on the ball.

My first experience in seeing patients on the ward was working in a cardiovascular unit where, in fact, we did treat people after myocardial infarction with linseed oil and this was part of a Nordic studies trial. The people who had already had a myocardial infarction did not greatly appreciate the linseed oil. They found it very unpalatable. So even if they had it while they were in hospital, because it could be poured in, in a way which you can do in hospital, I guess they were not going to take it when they got home.

One of my mentors as a student was Michael Oliver, who was a consultant in the wards that I was on as a young medical student. He has an important place in history, having set up the trial of clofibrate which was designed to run for 10 years, and which was a mammoth trial by any standards at all, and which after seven years, because of the excess deaths in the clofibrate branch of the trial, was

---

Address for correspondence: Dr John Ferguson, Medical Director, Prescription Pricing Authority, Bridge House, 152 Pilgrim Street, Newcastle Upon Tyne, NE1 6SN, UK.

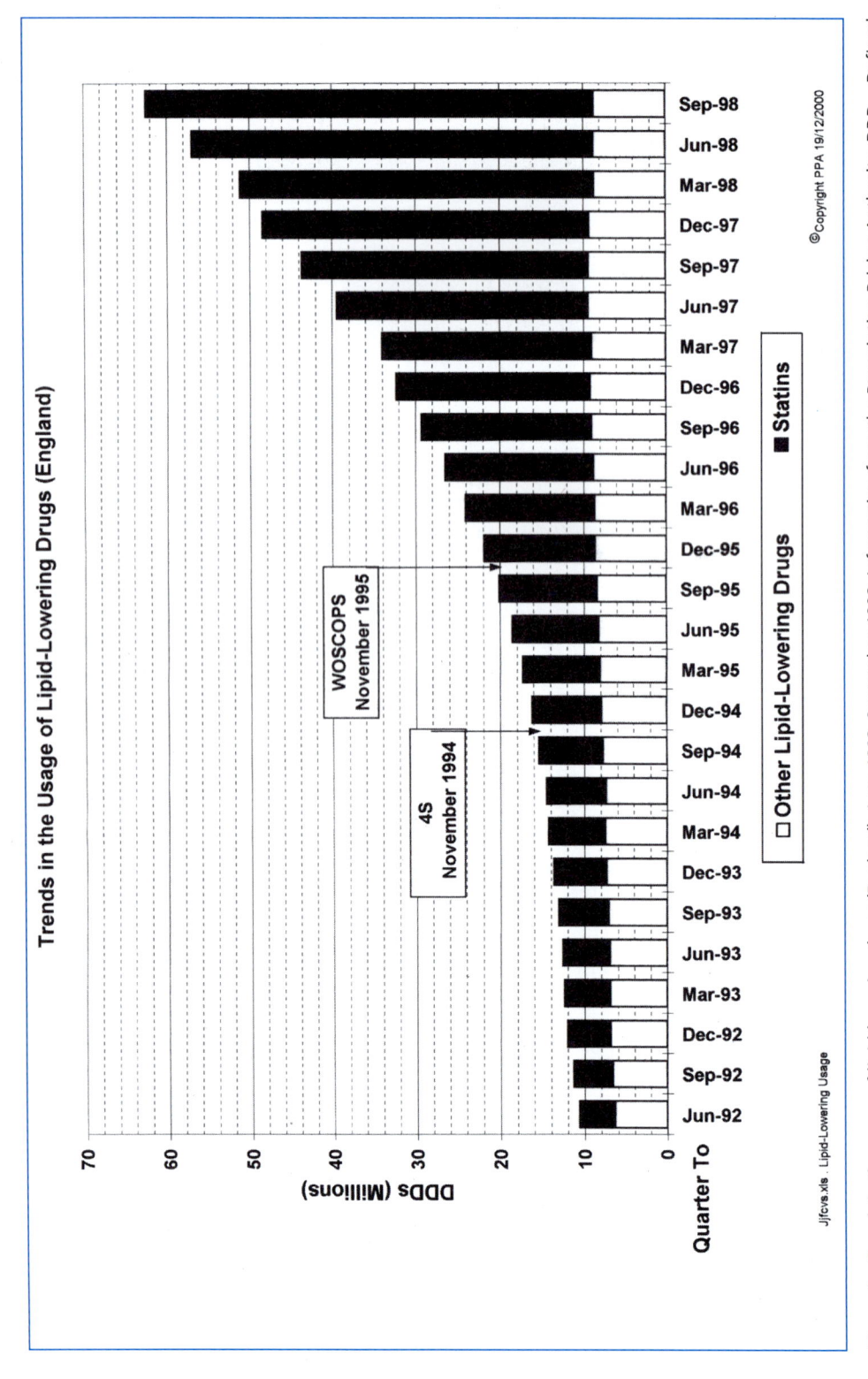

42 *Management of hypercholesterolaemia in primary health care*

Figure 1 Trends in the usage of lipid-lowering drugs (England). June 1992–September 1998. Information from the Prescription Pricing Authority. DDD = Defined drug doses. 4S = Scandinavian Simvastatin Survival Study. WOSCOPS = West of Scotland Coronary Prevention Study.

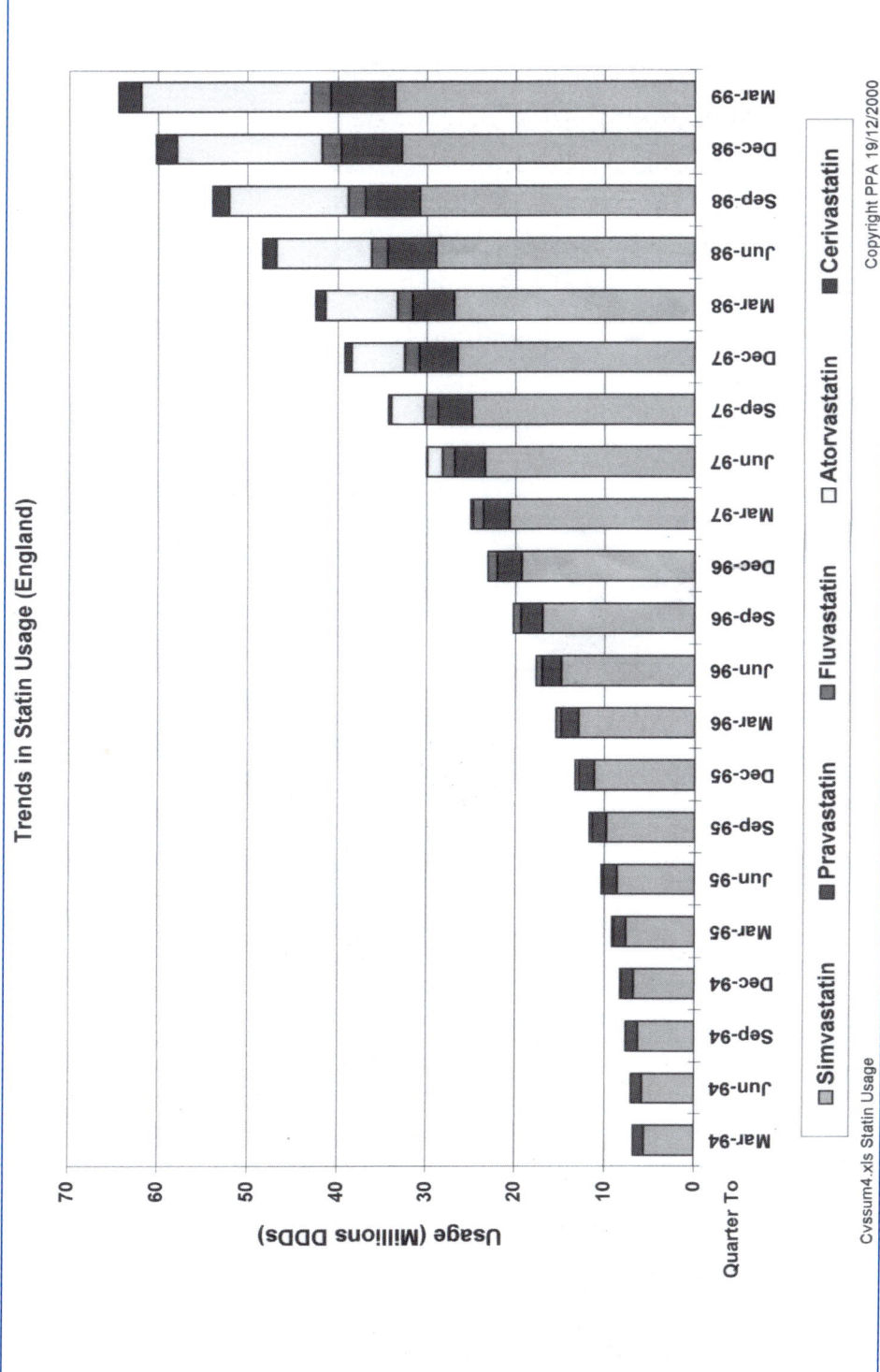

Figure 2 Trends in statin usage (England). March 1994–March 1999. Information from the Prescription Pricing Authority. DDD = Defined drug doses.

stopped prematurely. It was thought that these were non-cardiac deaths but nevertheless it was felt that the trial could not continue. After that Michael Oliver was very much against trying to alter cholesterol and it is interesting that, in his later career, he is now in favour of cholesterol management and trying to look after people's cholesterol levels. He has completed the whole circuit within his lifetime.

Besides the clinician's need to consider cholesterol, there is the problem of saturated and unsaturated fats. I remember that I used to get a hard time about 20 years ago from my wife about my butter consumption. But I'm an example of an n=1 trial because I was brought up on a large number of eggs from when I was a very small child and I've continued to have a high egg consumption ever since. When I was in Hong Kong, we used to get eggs from California which came from the Incredible Egg Company and these were just ordinary eggs as far as I could determine. But the net result of this was that when I was really driven to the wall, I decided that I would have my cholesterol test done and I discovered that I had one that was almost at the bottom of the normal range. And when I went back and I told my wife that, it meant that there has been silence ever since on this particular subject, and so from that point of view I can commend that to you as a means of countering persistent criticism.

One of the characteristics of cholesterol is that it is very easy biochemically to measure and so maybe one of the reasons why cholesterol was the thing that we latched onto. In the late 1980s there was a rise in the new patient testing which became very fashionable and was promoted by a large number of people. But I think one of the facts about medicine is that you do not tend to diagnose things you cannot treat and you do not treat things you cannot diagnose. And so for a long time we did not have any very good treatments and so therefore there was no great point in making the diagnosis. When we could diagnose the condition easily, we did not have anything very good to offer the patients. We had the ion exchange resins, we had the fibrates and, at the beginning of the 1990s, we were just beginning to see the statins. That is the background against which the last 10 or so years have developed. While it is easy to latch onto cholesterol we are dealing with a multi-factorial illness and so this sort of one-directional approach of concentrating on cholesterol is probably wrong.

Primary practice in England

Drug prescribing patterns

In this section I will attempt to demonstrate the trends and patterns of prescribing in this particular area which is based on the English GP prescribing database. Figure 1 shows that the fibrates remained relatively static during the 1990s, which is hardly surprising as there has been virtually no new work being done on them to engender any great interest. The growth is, of course, in the statins and you can see the effect of the Scandinavian Simvastin Survival Study and by other studies and the way in which they have taken off almost exponentially ever since. You could argue that we are rapidly reaching the stage where we need to consider putting them in the domestic water supply!

There have been some questions as to which statin. There is an argument now about whether statins are all basically the same. Is it a class effect and, therefore, you do not need to worry too much about which one you are going to use? Figure 2 shows that simvastatin has been the most successful of the statins to date. Pravastatin came in next but has never taken off to the same extent. Fluvastatin has really gone nowhere. Atorvastatin, as somebody has said, is the flavour of month, and Cerivastatin is there too. But you can see the way in which there has been recent growth in atorvastatin.

Figure 3 shows the standardised analysis of the 100 health authorities in England, and you can see that there is quite a variation in the total use of statins across the country and in fact there is an approximate 3.7-fold variation from the lowest to the highest usage. The messages from this figure are, first of all, that across the country simvastatin is number one in every health authority and at the time of these data (1997), in most health authorities, pravastatin was number two, though in one or two of them, atorvastatin was already

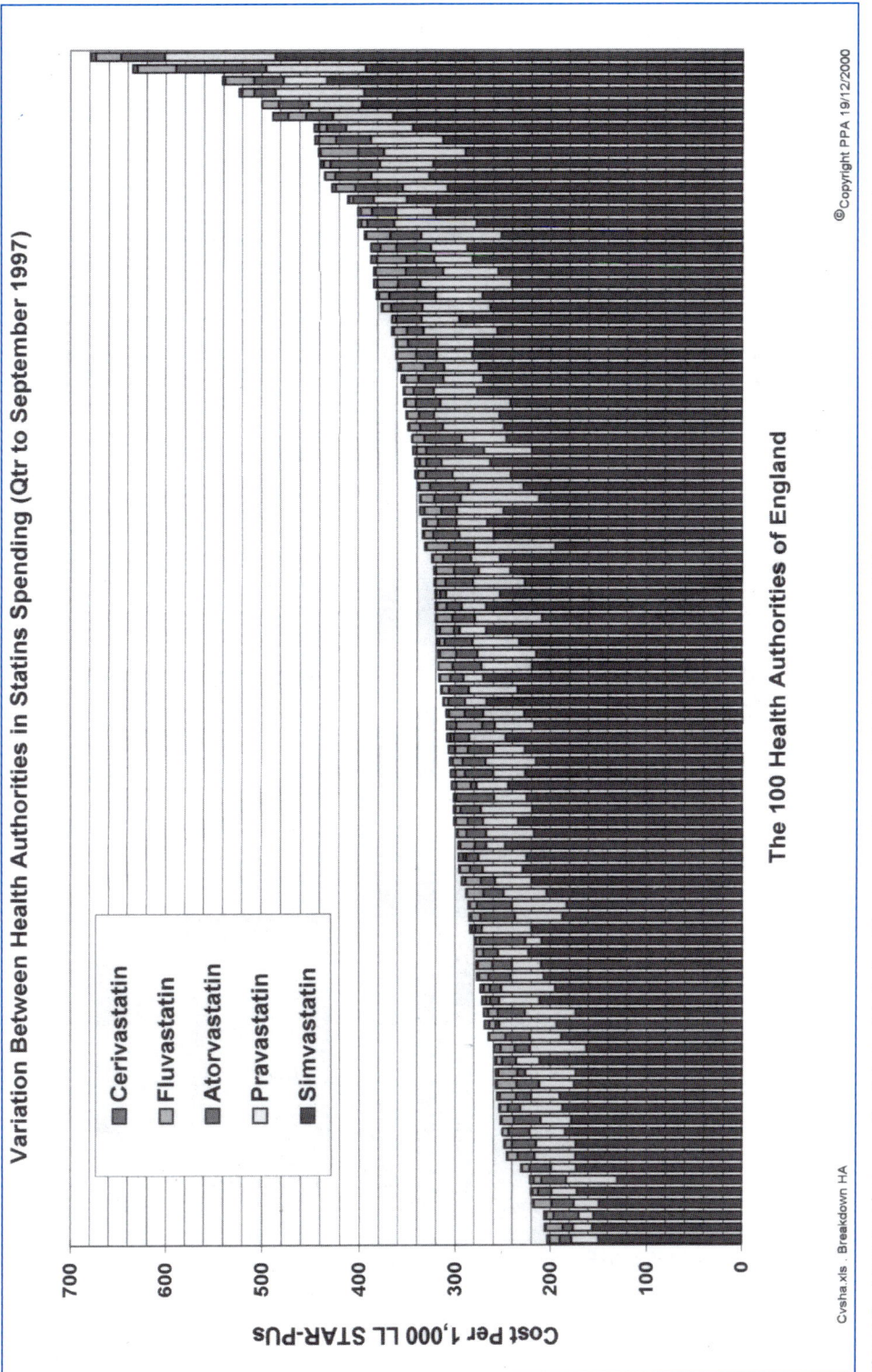

Figure 3 Variation between English Health Authorities in spending on statins (3rd quarter of 1997). Information from the Prescription Pricing Authority. LL-STAR-PUs = Lipid-lowering specific therapeutic group age- and sex-related prescribing units.

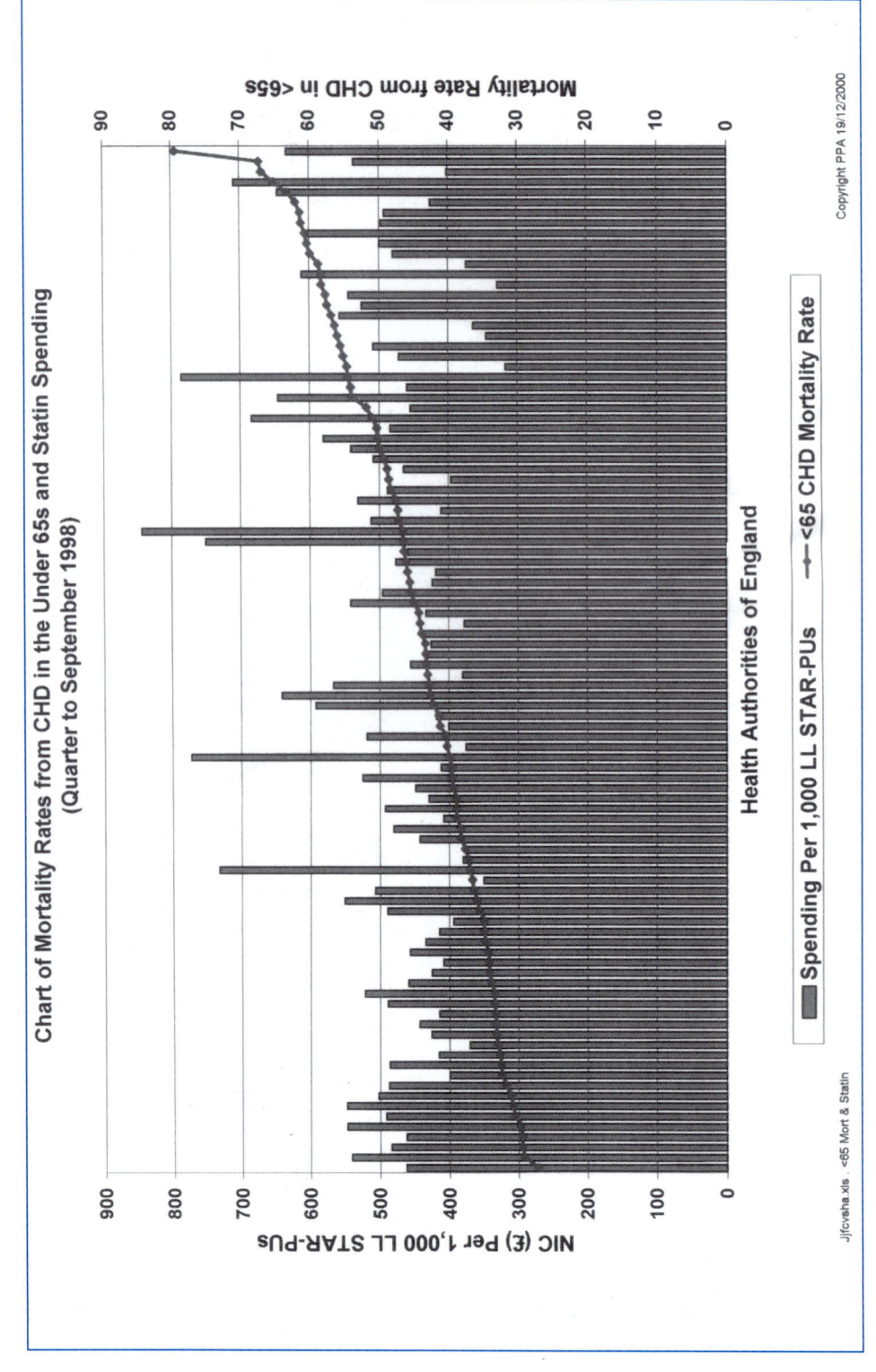

46 *Management of hypercholesterolaemia in primary health care*

Figure 4 Chart of mortality rates from CHD in under 65s and statin spending (3rd quarter of 1998). Information from the Prescription Pricing Authority. NIC = Net ingredient costs. LL-STAR-PUs = Lipid-lowering specific therapeutic group age- and sex-related prescribing units.

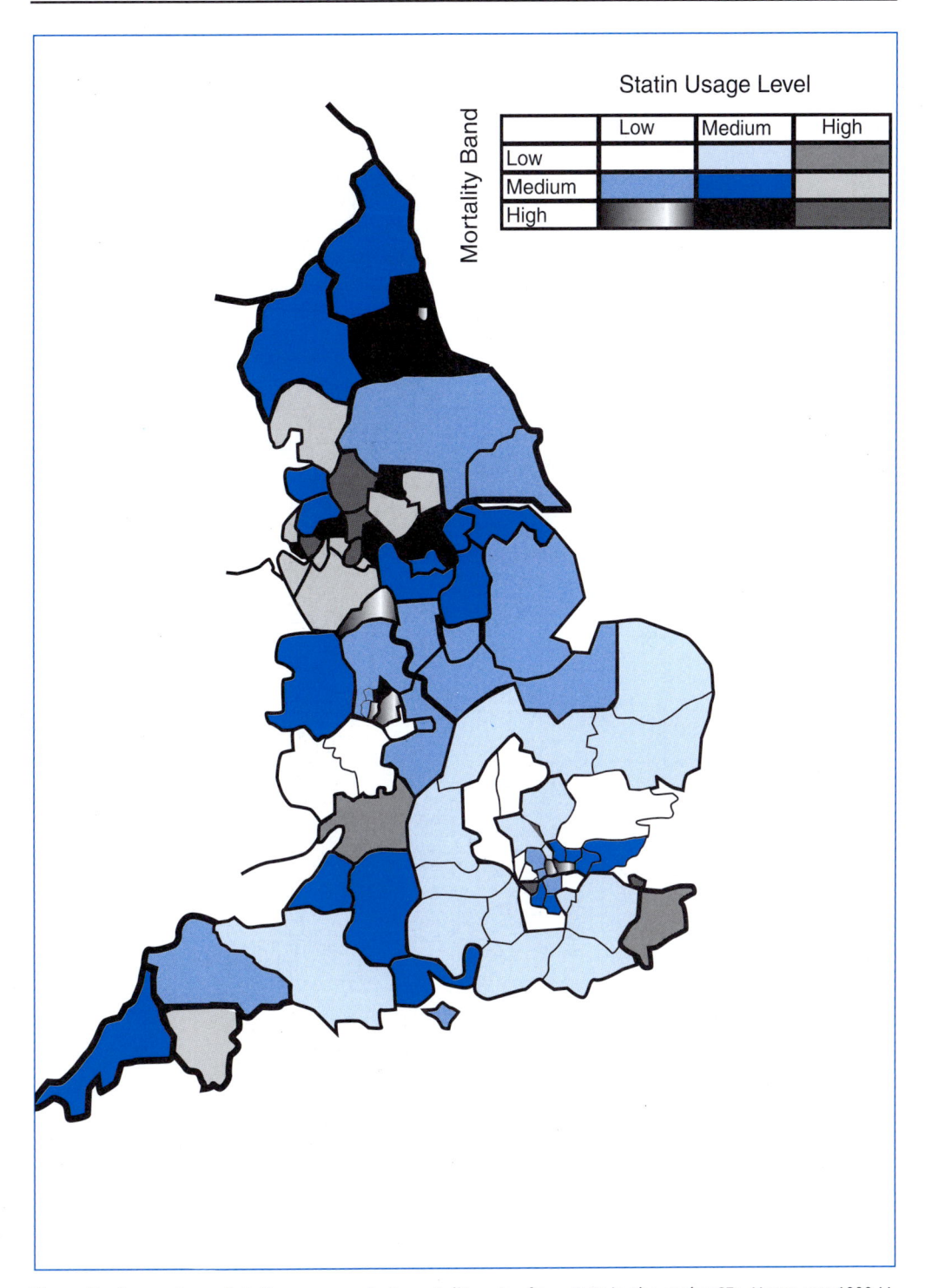

Figure 5 Comparison of statin usage against mortality rates from CHD in the under-65s. Usage per 1000 LL STAR-PUs (3rd quarter of 1997). Information from the Prescription Pricing Authority. LL-STAR-PUs = L:ipid-lowering specific therapeutic group age- and sex-related prescribing units.

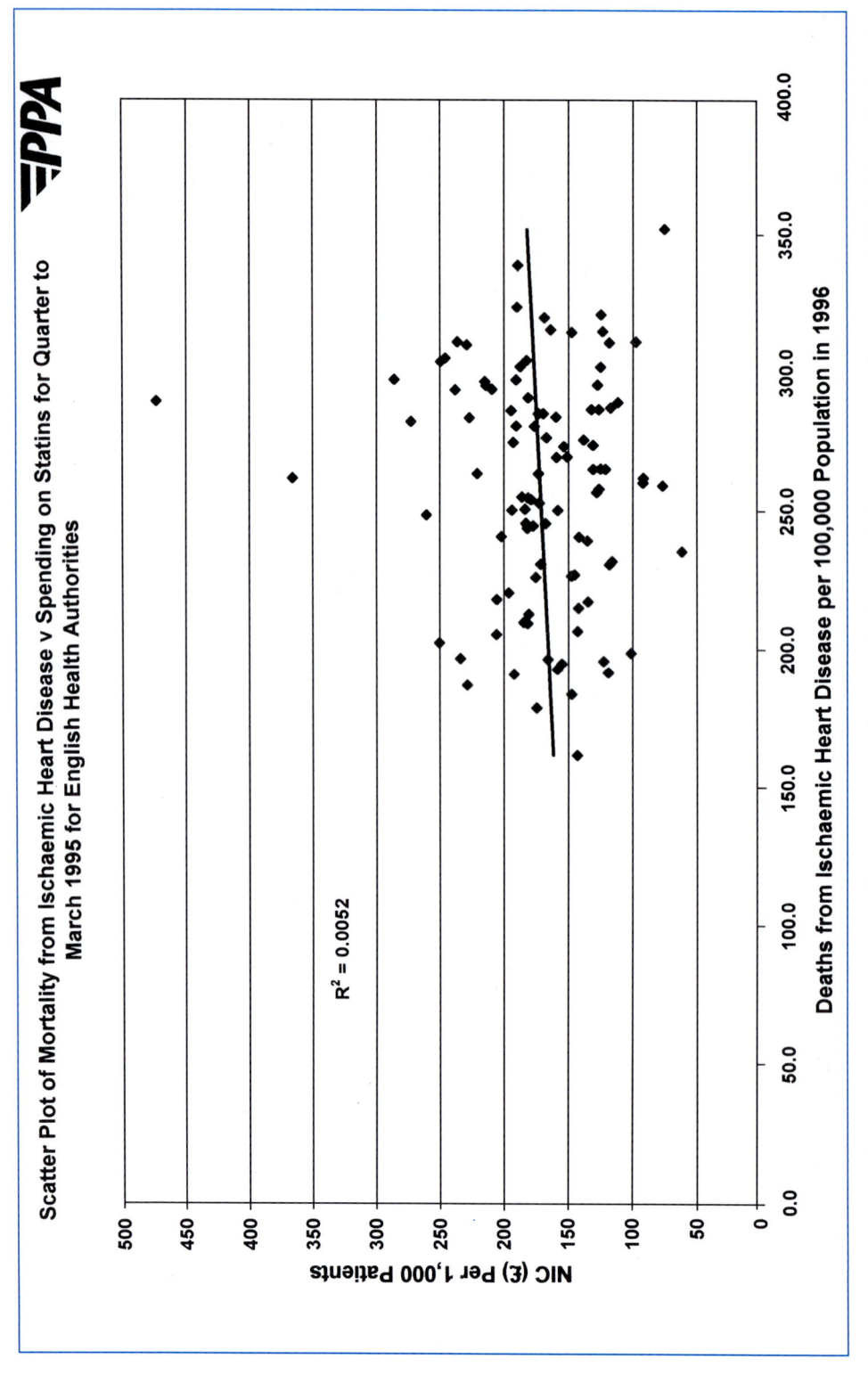

48 *Management of hypercholesterolaemia in primary health care*

Figure 6 Scatter plot of mortality from ischaemic heart disease versus spending on statins for English Health Authorities (1st quarter of 1995). Information from the Prescription Pricing Authority. NIC = Net ingredient costs.

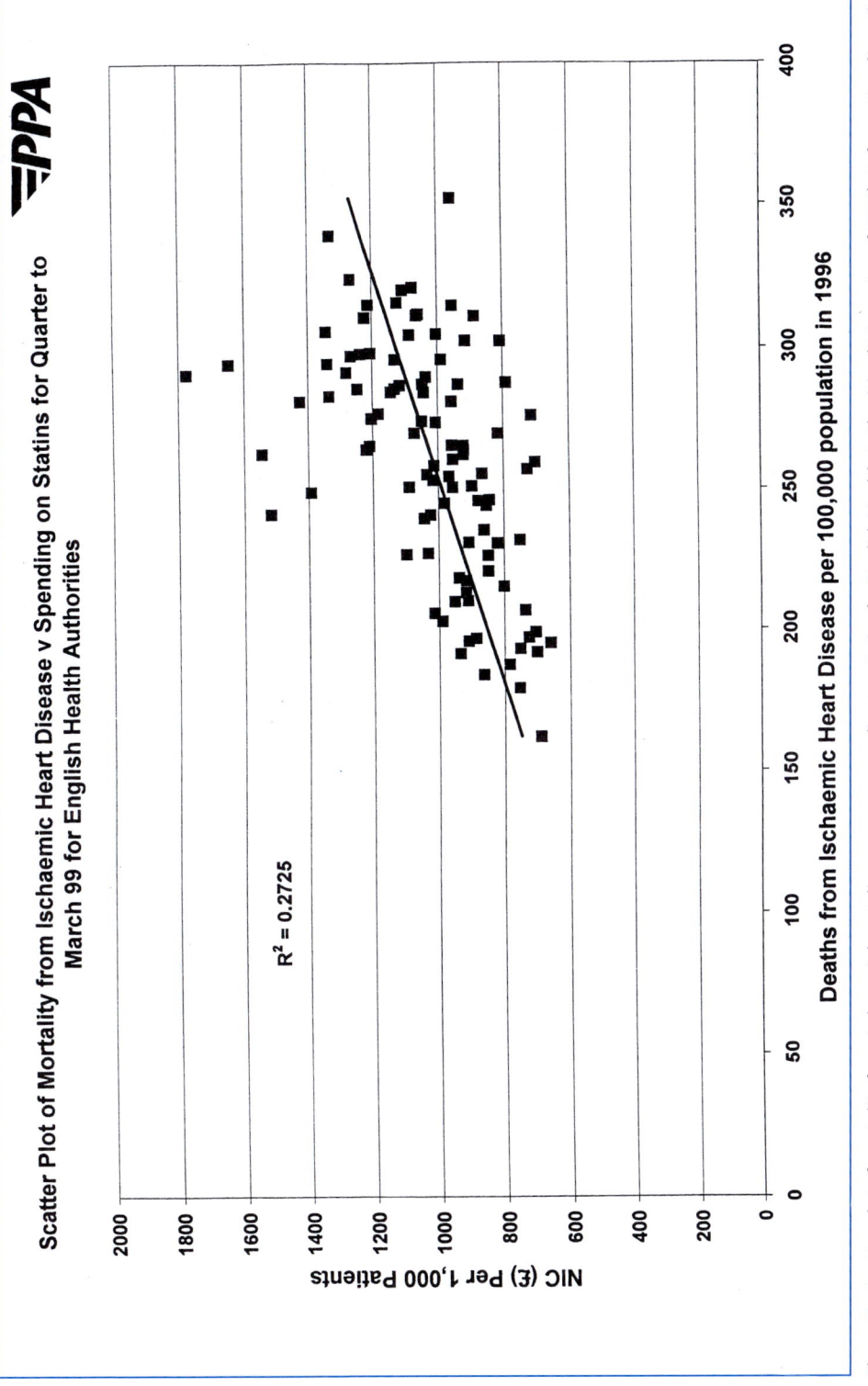

Figure 7 Scatter plot of mortality from ischaemic heart disease versus spending on statins for English Health Authorities (1st quarter of 1999). Information from the Prescription Pricing Authority. NIC = Net ingredient costs.

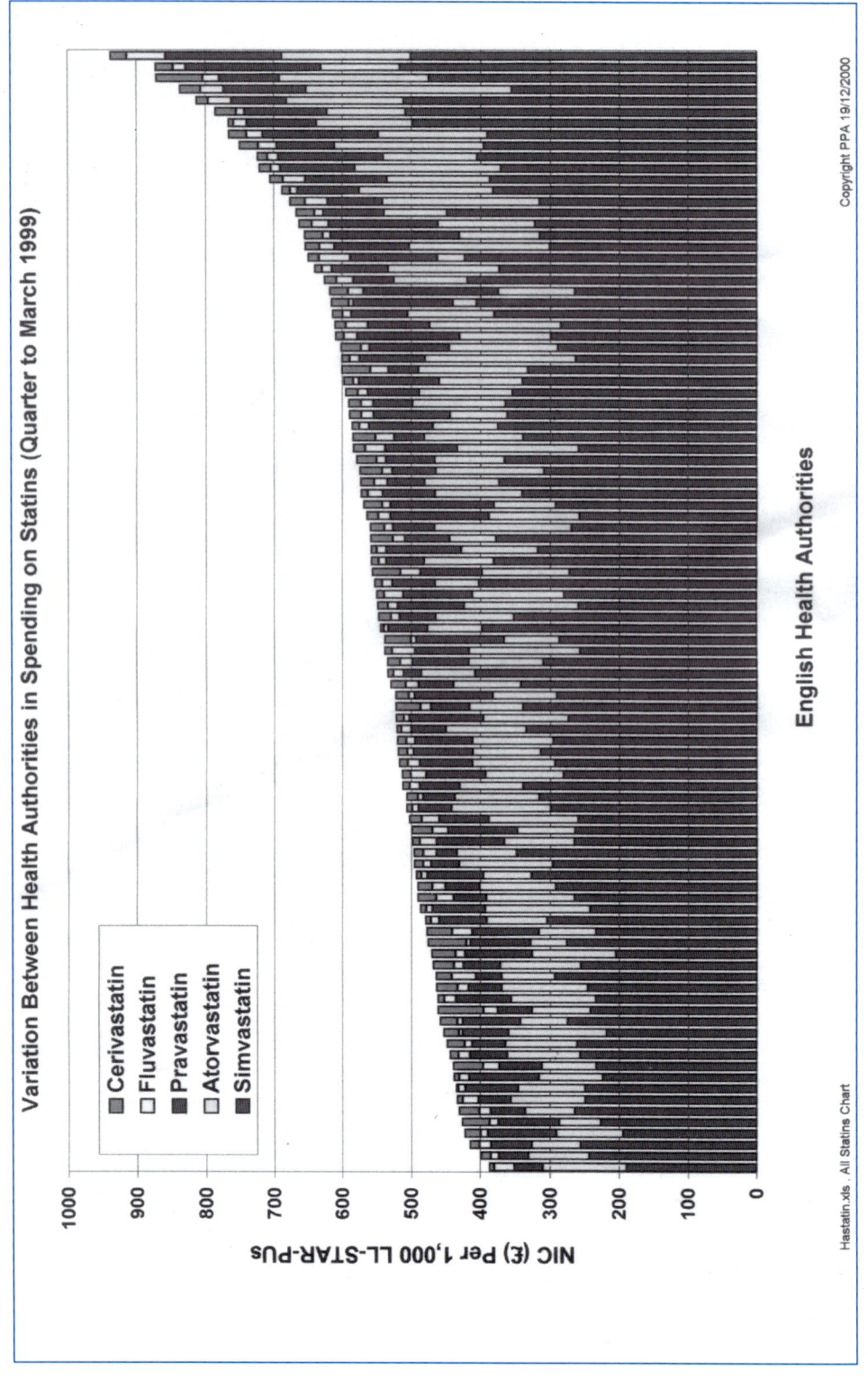

50 *Management of hypercholesterolaemia in primary health care*

Figure 8 Variation between health authorities in spending on statins (1st quarter of 1999). Information from the Prescription Pricing Authority. NIC = Net ingredient costs. LL-STAR-PUs = Lipid-lowering specific therapeutic group age- and sex-related prescribing units.

beginning to come in. But nobody has yet defined what is the correct level of prescribing.

If we try and compare the prescribing of statins along with the public health data on mortality from CHD then again it is not very clear that there is any real association across the country. Figure 4 shows the mortality rate of health authorities, and the actual spend on statins. Now the difficulty is that across the country there is a socio-economic spread by geographical region. The North is less healthy than the South. The old heavy industries are mainly in the North of the country. People who are less socially advantaged are in the North. There is more unemployment, there is more deprivation, there is more chronic illness, so you would expect to see more illness in the North of the country. When we try and plot these two things together, it is difficult once again to see a consistent pattern. Figure 5 shows a plot of these two different factors, using a simple 3 x 3 plot, to give the statin-spending against mortality across the whole of England.

If it was following some sort of logical pattern, you would like to think that there would be plenty of the lower/lower, medium/medium, and high/high linkage of spending and disease. It does not quite look like that. It is quite concerning that we do have some places where the mortality is high from cardiovascular disease yet the amount of statin prescribing is low. On the other hand, there are some areas where the mortality is low and the spending is high. It is very difficult to see why in some areas there is perhaps too much prescribing in comparison with morbidity and mortality – and the reverse is also true. This is for under-65s and a very similar picture is shown for the over-65s, so there is nothing very much to show by looking at different age groups, as the same mismatches apply.

There is a real scatter as Figure 6 shows. If you try to correlate ischemic heart disease with statin spending there is no association at all. In 1995 you can see the line is pretty nearly horizontal and the spots are all over the place. So with the passage of time, has anything improved? Figure 7 shows that the scatter is getting less and the line is becoming improved. If we actually look again at the 100 health authorities in 1999 (Figure 8), you can see both that there is more prescribing and that the variation has been reduced from 3.7 times to 2.6 times, with less variation from the lowest to the highest health authorities. Simvastatin is still number 1 in all the English health authorities, but atorvastatin is coming in as number 2 in a large number of the health authorities and in this context is displacing pravastatin.

Prescribing and prevention

But, again, who are prescribing at the right level? I showed these data recently to cardiologists working in hospital and they said that GPs had 'got it all wrong' and that prescribing should be even higher. However, we may be just throwing statins at a problem that we have not very clearly defined. I think that though these figures show that the prescribing of statins has improved, it leaves some fundamental questions. We still are treating a biochemical diagnosis, that is a high cholesterol level. We recognise that across the country we have no clear association with disease. We do not know what the correct level is anyway.

The other real problem is, are we going to try and actually treat people for primary prevention or secondary prevention? In simple terms, do you start treating the diagnosis as soon as you have identified it, which means you may go on treating them for a very long time, or do you treat only those who are at greatest risk – and you treat them, of course, for a shorter period of time? In public health, epidemiology terms, it is actually better value for money to treat people for secondary prevention and not primary prevention. We see prescriptions which are written across the country and we know whether these are for men or for women. Does it come as a surprise to you, that across the country the ratio of prescriptions for statins are 55% for men and 45% for women? Does that actually fit what you expect should be the case, what would be rational? Because if you start looking at risk tables, whether they are Sheffield (UK) risk tables or New Zealand risk tables or others, it means looking at treating women who are over the age of 70, who have probably got hypertension, and who may have diabetes. I do not believe that half the population on statins in this country have those degrees of risk. It is my belief that we need to do a lot more to target the use of these drugs to get the best results.

Need for a consistent health message
What are we going to do now? What is the next stage? There are aspirations for the new British National Health Service (NHS) and we have got the National Institute for Clinical Excellence (NICE) providing guidance, and there is the Commission for Health Improvement to monitor the health service. We have the new Clinical Governance, a sort of clinical audit to try and tell us what we should be doing in the NHS. National Service Framework for Coronary Heart Disease has recently been set up. So we are not short of advice. The problem is whether we have consistent advice. As has already been suggested sometimes these targets are actually set at values that will be achieved anyway, regardless of what happens. We must look at all the risk factors. It seems to me that the one risk factor that is still the highest single risk factor is not cholesterol but smoking. Obesity has been discussed in this meeting. There is a range of risk factors. Some calculations put the effect of serum cholesterol at about 12.5% of the whole.

The important thing is to try and concentrate on the risk factors that are actually going to make the difference and to concentrate our message on one thing at a time. For my money, it has got to be smoking and you cannot tell people they must stop smoking and that they must lose weight at the same time, because these two messages are mutually contradictory. If you are going to talk about lifestyles, then you have to understand what motivates people to do the things they do and you must actually take this on board if people are to take these messages seriously. There has to be a consistent message and as emphasised by others in the field. I cannot help but agree that across the primary health care teams we have all to work together with a consistent message. A lot of the health advice is not just given by doctors but also given by health visitors. It is a sad reflection on the present state of affairs that dietitians are not involved to any great extent in primary care. I would like to see more dietitians out in the community.

Alternative treatments
We have got an interesting situation that until recently the government has always refused to consider giving any treatment that would help people to stop smoking. It has been only in the last little while that they have not blacklisted the latest nicotine replacement therapies which have got some proven marginal benefit. But their argument in the past has always been that if you can afford to smoke, you can afford to stop smoking and buy your nicotine replacement therapy. There is no other illness, and no other treatment, within medicine that I know of where you actually say to people you should buy it yourself for your own self-inflicted condition. So I think there is a rather bizarre argument around nicotine replacement and I guess that the government's attitude is changing because we have recently seen that a new anti-smoking treatment, Zyban, is going to be licensed for use on the NHS. You could, I suppose, say that similar arguments apply to the role of Benecol, and that if it is proven to be useful then perhaps it also should be available on the NHS for people who need it.

Dietary cholesterol as a cardiac risk factor: myth or reality? Ed Anthony R Leeds, Juliet Gray. ©2001. Smith-Gordon. Printed in UK.

6   Eggs, dietary cholesterol and cardiac risk – a US perspective

Donald J. McNamara

Egg Nutrition Center, Washington, DC 20036, USA

For 30 years dietary recommendations in the United States included restricting dietary cholesterol to less than 300 mg per day, a recommendation based on results from animal studies, epidemiological surveys, and clinical feeding trials.

Animal studies are compromised by two factors: species variability in response to dietary cholesterol, and the non-human-like plasma lipoprotein profiles of most animals. Epidemiological data analyzed by simple correlations suggest that dietary cholesterol is related to CVD incidence whereas multiple correlation analyses indicate that dietary cholesterol is not associated with increased CVD risk. Meta-analyses of clinical feeding studies show that the average plasma cholesterol response to dietary cholesterol is 0.00062 mmol/l (0.024 mg/dl) per mg/day cholesterol. The data indicate that dietary cholesterol raises both atherogenic LDL and anti-atherogenic HDL cholesterol concentrations with little effect on the LDL:HDL ratio, a determinant of CVD risk.

The available data fail to validate the need for dietary cholesterol restrictions to lower CHD risk. This is especially true for eggs which are low in saturated fat and provide a variety of essential and functional nutrients.

Introduction

For the past 30 years conventional wisdom has held that intake of cholesterol from foods increases plasma cholesterol levels and therefore increases cardiovascular disease (CVD) risk. High cholesterol foods such as eggs are not only restricted in therapeutic plasma-cholesterol-lowering diets but limits are also often recommended for the general healthy population. The basis for dietary cholesterol restrictions was derived from animal studies, epidemiological surveys and clinical feeding studies [1, 2]. From a public health perspective it seemed prudent, based on the available data, to take a precautionary approach and assume the worst, even if the information relating CVD risk and dietary cholesterol was uncertain. The problem is that, while these early recommendations were best estimates at the time based on relatively weak evidence, over the years they are perceived as being based on sound scientific evidence, and rarely does anyone question the rationale of the restriction. When a dietary restriction reaches that level of wide acceptance, as in the case of dietary cholesterol and egg consumption, it is no longer the responsibility of those making the risk claims to prove the validity of the assertion, but rather it is up to those denying the accusation to prove that it is not true ('reverse onus').

The theoretical relationship between eggs,

Address for correspondence: Dr Donald J McNamara, Executive Director, Egg Nutrition Center, 1050 17th St., NW, Suite 560, Washington DC 20036, USA.

dietary cholesterol and CVD risk is based on two facts and one assumption. Fact one is that an increased plasma cholesterol level, specifically plasma low-density-lipoprotein (LDL) cholesterol, is related to an increased risk of CVD. Assumption one is that dietary cholesterol raises plasma cholesterol levels which are associated with increased CVD risk. Fact two is that eggs are a concentrated source of cholesterol in the diet that contributes approximately one-third of the daily cholesterol intake [3].

The rationale for assuming the validity of these theoretical relationships was based on three criteria: animal studies indicating that dietary cholesterol raises blood cholesterol; epidemiological relationships between dietary cholesterol and CVD incidence, and clinical trials showing a positive correlation between cholesterol intakes and plasma cholesterol levels. These relationships justified dietary cholesterol and egg restrictions 30 years ago, but today there is substantial evidence that this seemingly rational relationship is in fact not real and that cholesterol in food is unrelated to CVD risk [4–6].

Lines of evidence

Animal studies

Cholesterol-feeding studies in animal models have resulted in mixed results and are highly dependent upon two factors: the species of animal being studied and the amount of cholesterol being fed. Some animal species are hypersensitive to the plasma cholesterol effects of dietary cholesterol while others are resistant to any effects of dietary cholesterol. To further complicate interpretation of animal studies, researchers often use extreme intakes of cholesterol to study relationships between hypercholesterolemia and atherosclerosis, and then make conclusions regarding effects of dietary factors on plasma lipoprotein-cholesterol levels. Feeding levels of 1.5–3.0 g cholesterol per 1000 kcal has little relevance to effects of physiological intakes on CVD risk. Finally, extrapolation of animal studies to human health is complicated by the fact that animal models have distinct plasma lipoprotein profiles which are dramatically different from the profile found in humans.

Epidemiological surveys

In the 1970s and 1980s a number of reports indicated a significant positive relationship between dietary cholesterol and CVD incidence [7, 8]. In almost every case the relationship was based on a simple correlation between dietary cholesterol and CVD rates; however, in these same studies there was a positive and statistically more significant relationship between dietary saturated fat intake and CVD incidence. These studies also show that dietary cholesterol and saturated fat are highly correlated to each other which complicates interpretation of the data.

In the late 1980s and 1990s most epidemiological surveys utilized multiple regression techniques in data analysis in order to account for the co-linearity of dietary variables, and these studies consistently report no significant relationship between dietary cholesterol and CVD rates [9–15]. There have been no epidemiological survey data showing a significant relationship between dietary cholesterol and CVD rates when the data are adjusted for the co-linearity of saturated fatty acid calories. Data from a number of case-control studies of diet and CVD rates were summarized by Ravnskov [16] and indicated that the difference in cholesterol intake between cases and controls averaged 16 mg/day per 1000 kcal. This intake difference occurred in a metabolic system with an overall daily cholesterol mass input (dietary and newly synthesized) and output (excretion and metabolism to bile acids) of over 1000 mg/day [17]. It hardly seems feasible that this small difference in dietary cholesterol could account for the difference in CVD incidence.

Eggs represent a high cholesterol food which is low in saturated fat and as such would be predicted, based on the evidence presented above, not to be significantly related to CVD risk. Data from the Framingham Heart Study indicated no significant relationship between egg consumption and either plasma cholesterol levels or heart disease rates [18]. Similar findings have been reported from other epidemiological surveys [19–22] and the overall findings indicate that egg consumption is unrelated to CVD risk. The most definitive study to date on the relationship between egg consumption and heart disease risk was reported by Hu et al [22] from two prospective studies, the 80 082 participants in the Nurses' Health Study and the 37 851 males in the Health Professionals Follow-Up Study. The data indicated that the risk for CVD was the same whether the participants consumed less than one egg a week or more than one egg a day (Table 1). This lack of a relationship was true for normocholesterolemics and hypercholesterolemics, and independent of other dietary and physiological factors. The only sub-set exhibiting a significant relationship between egg intake and CVD was individuals with diabetes.

Analysis of international data for per capita egg consumption and CVD mortality rates showed a negative relationship [6] with Japan, Mexico, France and Spain having the highest per capita consumption levels and the lowest rates of CVD mortality. In Japan, per capita egg consumption approached an egg a day yet CVD death rates are the lowest of any industrialized country. Clearly the cross-cultural data do not provide any evidence in support of a positive relationship between egg consumption and CVD incidence.

The evidence from epidemiological surveys, both case-control and prospective, indicates that there is no significant independent relationship between dietary cholesterol, or eggs, and CVD risk [6, 23]. In 1989 a study suggested that with extremely high intakes of cholesterol CVD risk was increased [7]; however, in this study cholesterol intake in the high-risk group exceeded 1000 mg/day [24], suggesting an extreme intake of animal products, and a correspondingly low intake of fruits and vegetables. With this dietary pattern it is not surprising that there is an increased risk of CVD due to low fiber intake [25–28], low B vitamin intake [29–31] and low antioxidant intake [32–35], all factors related to increased risk of CVD. The unresolved issue is whether subjects with the most extreme intakes of dietary cholesterol were at increased CVD risk from what they were consuming, or at risk due to the absence of sufficient intakes of nutrients associated with CVD risk reduction. Until this question is resolved it cannot be shown that dietary cholesterol per se is a causal factor in CVD, especially when there is a large body of evidence indicative of no association between cholesterol intake and CVD risk.

Clinical feeding trials

Since 1960 there have been over 160 cholesterol-feeding studies in more than 3500 study subjects [4, 36–39]. There has also been a number of analyses of these studies to determine the average plasma lipoprotein cholesterol response to dietary cholesterol and the associated dietary and physiological variables which impact on this response [4, 36, 40–43]. The various studies have all come to a similar conclusion, a 100 mg/day change in dietary cholesterol will change plasma total cholesterol levels by an average of 2.4 mg/dl. This small effect on plasma cholesterol levels explains why, in the early studies of the effects of dietary factors on plasma lipids, it was necessary to feed subjects amounts of cholesterol as high as 4000 mg/day in order to achieve measurable changes in plasma cholesterol levels [4]. Studies using more physiological ranges of intakes (addition of 200–400 mg/day or of one to two eggs per day) consistently report little or no measurable changes in plasma total cholesterol levels [44–49].

A basic assumption in the dietary-cholesterol plasma-cholesterol heart-disease relationship hypothesis has been that any increase in plasma total cholesterol is associated with an increase in CVD risk. It could therefore be argued that, even though dietary cholesterol has only a small effect on plasma cholesterol levels, any lowering achieved by egg restrictions would be beneficial. In a detailed analysis of data from controlled feed-

Table 1 Egg consumption and heart disease risk.

Weekly egg consumption	Coronary heart disease relative risk (95% CI)	
	Men (n=37 851)	Women (n=80 082)
<1	1.0	1.0
1	1.06 (0.88–1.27)	0.82 (0.67–1.00)
2–4	1.12 (0.95–1.33)	0.99 (0.82–1.18)
5–6	0.90 (0.63–1.27)	0.95 (0.60–1.13)
≥7	1.08 (0.79–1.48)	0.82 (0.60–1.13)
P for trend	0.75	0.95

Data from Hu et al [22]. CI = confidence interval.

Table 2 Egg consumption and plasma lipoprotein cholesterol levels.

Cholesterol (mmol/l)	Baseline diet	Baseline + egg/day
Total	5.43	5.56
LDL	3.36	3.47
HDL	1.29	1.32
LDL:HDL ratio	2.61	2.63

ing studies, Clarke et al [41] reported that dietary cholesterol increased not only plasma levels of atherogenic LDL cholesterol but also increased the anti-atherogenic HDL cholesterol levels. Similar data have been reported from an analysis of all published cholesterol-feeding studies [4] and indicated that a 100 mg/day change in dietary cholesterol increases plasma cholesterol by 2.4 mg/dl, LDL cholesterol by 1.9 mg/dl and HDL cholesterol by 0.4 mg/dl. A number of studies have reported the finding that dietary cholesterol does not alter the LDL:HDL ratio [44–48], a significant determinant of CVD risk. As shown in Table 2, adding an egg a day to the diet has little effect on the LDL:HDL cholesterol ratio.

Why not restrict eggs just to be safe?

It is assumed that egg restrictions do not have any negative consequences and therefore, to be on the safe side, limitations are harmless and may possibly benefit some individuals who are hyper-responders to dietary cholesterol [4]. But is this really true? Eggs are an affordable source of high quality protein and contain a wide variety of essential vitamins and minerals. More importantly, eggs have a high nutrient density relative to the caloric content which can play an important role in weight maintenance. In addition, recent studies have been finding beneficial nutrients in eggs which, due to the composition of the egg, have high bioavailability.

There is good evidence that the risks of cataracts and age-related macular degeneration are related to low intakes of the carotenoid xanthophylls lutein and zeaxanthin which are known to accumulate in the macular region of the eye [50]. Studies by Handelman et al [51] have shown that egg feeding significantly increased plasma levels of lutein and zeaxanthin. Consistent with this observation, data from the Beaver Dam Eye Study cohort indicated a significant negative relationship between egg consumption and nuclear cataract risk [52].

Eggs also serve as a good source of choline, a newly recognized essential nutrient important in brain development and memory [53–55]. Studies in animals indicate that choline plays essentials roles in the development of brain function and in memory. Choline supplementation during gestation in rats leads to augmentation of spatial memory in adulthood and studies indicate that dietary choline treatment can render new long-term memories less susceptible to disruption following training. The National Academy of Sciences recently recognized choline as an essential nutrient with a recommended adequate intake (AI) for men, women and children. For adults the AI values are 425 mg per day for women and 550 mg per day for men. Pregnant and lactating women are advised to increase their choline intakes. A large egg has 215 mg of choline, almost 50% of the recommended AI for adults, and eggs can readily serve as an excellent source of choline for pregnant and lactating women.

Conclusions and comment

The evidence that dietary cholesterol, and high cholesterol foods like eggs, contribute to CVD risk is very weak, and the majority of epidemiological studies find a null relationship between cholesterol in foods and CVD incidence. The observation that feeding gram quantities of cholesterol measurably increased plasma cholesterol levels was considered sufficient evidence of potential risk to warrant dietary cholesterol restrictions; however, studies have shown that physiological amounts of dietary cholesterol have only a small effect on plasma cholesterol levels, and that the increase occurs not only in the plasma LDL cholesterol fraction, but also in the HDL cholesterol, with no significant effect on the LDL:HDL cholesterol ratio.

The precautionary principle advises that

when risk is uncertain it is prudent to assume the worst. The complication, however, is that when there is sufficient evidence indicating an absence of risk, it is almost impossible to reverse the longstanding condemnation. For over 30 years cholesterol has been considered a major dietary evil, and the egg became the icon for both dietary and blood cholesterol. The re-education of the health community and the public regarding the absence of a health risk associated with egg consumption, and its replacement with an understanding of the health benefits associated with including eggs in a healthy, nutritious diet, will be a slow and tedious process.

Is egg consumption associated with hypercholesterolemia and cardiovascular disease? The evidence says no. This is a myth whose time has passed. It is now time to address those dietary factors that do play a role in heart disease risk, with attention to nutrients which increase risk and nutrients which reduce risk. With today's understanding of the multiplicity of dietary factors involved in health promotion and disease prevention, it is time to move past the 'bad food' approach in patient education and provide the public with the knowledge and understanding of what constitutes a healthy diet and the old fashioned concepts of balance, variety and moderation.

References

1. American Heart Association. Diet and heart disease. Dallas: American Heart Association, 1968.
2. Grundy SM, Bilheimer D, Blackburn H, Brown WV, Kwiterovich Jr, PO, Mattson F, Schonfeld G, Weidman WH. Rationale of the diet-heart statement of the American Heart Association. Circulation 1982:65, 839A–54A.
3. Federation of American Societies for Experimental Biology. Report on nutrition monitoring in the United States. Volume 1. Washington DC: US Government Printing Office, 1995.
4. McNamara DJ. The impact of egg limitations on coronary heart disease risk: Do the numbers add up? J Am Coll Nutr 2000:19, 540S–48S.
5. McNamara DJ. Eggs, dietary cholesterol and heart disease risk: an international perspective. In: Sim JS, Nakai S, Guenter W, eds. Egg nutrition and biotechnology. New York: CABI Publishing, 1999; 55–63.
6. McNamara DJ. Dietary cholesterol and atherosclerosis. Biochim Biophys Acta 2000. In press.
7. Stamler J, Shekelle R. Dietary cholesterol and human coronary heart disease. The epidemiological evidence. Arch Pathol Lab Med 1988:112, 1032–40.
8. Stamler J. Population studies. In: Levy R, Rifkind B, Dennis B, Ernst N, eds. Nutrition, lipids, and coronary heart disease. New York: Raven Press, 1979; 25–88.
9. Ascherio A, Rimm EB, Giovannucci EL, Spiegelman D, Stampfer M, Willett WC. Dietary fat and risk of coronary heart disease in men: Cohort follow up study in the United States. BMJ 1996:313, 84–90.
10. Hu FB, Stampfer MJ, Manson JE, Rimm E, Colditz GA, Rosner BA, Hennekens CH, Willett WC. Dietary fat intake and the risk of coronary heart disease in women. New Engl J Med 1997:337, 1491–9.
11. Millen BE, Franz MM, Quatromoni PA, Gagnon DR, Sonnenberg LM, Ordovas JM, Wilson PWF, Schaefer EJ, Cupples LA. Diet and plasma lipids in women. 1. Macronutrients and plasma total and low-density lipoprotein cholesterol in women: The Framingham nutrition studies. J Clin Epidemiol 1996:49, 657–63.
12. Pietinen P, Ascherio A, Korhonen P, Hartman AM, Willett WC, Albanes D, Virtamo J. Intake of fatty acids and risk of coronary heart disease in a cohort of Finnish men – The Alpha-Tocopherol, Beta-Carotene Cancer Prevention Study. Am J Epidemiol 1997:145, 876–87.
13. Hegsted DM, Ausman LM. Diet, alcohol and coronary heart disease in men. J Nutr 1988:118, 1184–9.
14. Esrey KL, Joseph L, Grover SA. Relationship between dietary intake and coronary heart disease mortality: Lipid Research Clinics Prevalence Follow-up Study. J Clin Epidemiol 1996:49, 211–16.
15. Kromhout D, Menotti A, Bloemberg B, Aravanis C, Blackburn H, Buzina R, Dontas AS, Fidanza F, Giampaoli S, Jansen A. Dietary saturated and trans fatty acids and cholesterol and 25-year mortality from coronary heart disease: the Seven Countries Study. Prev Med 1995:24, 308–15.
16. Ravnskov U. Quotation bias in reviews of the diet-heart idea. J Clin Epidemiol 1995:48, 713–19.
17. McNamara DJ. Effects of fat-modified diets on cholesterol and lipoprotein metabolism. Annu Rev Nutr 1987:7, 273–90.
18. Dawber TR, Nickerson RJ, Brand FN, Pool J. Eggs, serum cholesterol, and coronary heart disease. Am J Clin Nutr 1982:36, 617–25.
19. Toeller M, Buyken AE, Heitkamp G, Scherbaum WA, Krans HMJ, Fuller JH, Group EICS. Associa-

tions of fat and cholesterol intake with serum lipid levels and cardiovascular disease: The EURODIAB IDDM Complications Study. Exp Clin Endocrinol Diabetes 1999:107, 512–21.
20 Fraser GE. Diet and coronary heart disease: beyond dietary fats and low-density-lipoprotein cholesterol. Am J Clin Nutr 1994:59, 1117S–23S.
21 Gramenzi A, Gentile A, Fasoli M, Negri E, Parazzini F, La Vecchia C. Association between certain foods and risk of acute myocardial infarction in women. BMJ 1990:300, 771–3.
22 Hu FB, Stampfer MJ, Rimm EB, Manson JE, Ascherio A, Colditz GA, Rosner BA, Spiegelman D, Speizer FE, Sacks FR, Hennekens CH, Willett WC. A prospective study of egg consumption and risk of cardiovascular disease in men and women. JAMA 1999:281, 1387–94.
23 Kritchevsky SB, Kritchevsky D. Egg consumption and coronary heart disease: An epidemiologic overview. J Am Coll Nutr 2000:19, 549S–55S.
24 Shekelle RB, Stamler J. Dietary cholesterol and ischaemic heart disease. Lancet 1989:i, 1177–8.
25 Pietinen P, Rimm EB, Korhonen P, Hartman AM, Willett WC, Albanes D, Virtamo J. Intake of dietary fiber and risk of coronary heart disease in a cohort of Finnish men – The Alpha-Tocopherol, Beta-Carotene Cancer Prevention Study. Circulation 1996:94, 2720–27.
26 Rimm EB, Willett WC, Hu FB, Sampson L, Colditz GA, Manson JE, Hennekens C, Stampfer MJ. Folate and vitamin B6 from diet and supplements in relation to risk of coronary heart disease among women. JAMA 1998:279, 359–64.
27 Anderson JW, Hanna TJ, Peng XJ, Kryscio RJ. Whole grain foods and heart disease risk. J Am Coll Nutr 2000:19, 291S–9S.
28 Stampfer MJ, Hu FB, Manson JE, Rimm EB, Willett WC. Primary prevention of coronary heart disease in women through diet and lifestyle. New Engl J Med 2000:343, 16–22.
29 Wilcken DEL, Wilcken B. B vitamins and homocysteine in cardiovascular disease and aging. Ann NY Acad Sci 1998:854, 361–70.
30 Robinson K. Homocysteine, B vitamins, and risk of cardiovascular disease. Heart 2000:83, 127–30.
31 Seshadri N, Robinson K. Homocysteine, B vitamins, and coronary artery disease. Med Clin North Am 2000:84, 215–37.
32 Gaziano JM. Antioxidants in cardiovascular disease: Randomized trials. Nutr Rev 1996:54, 175–7.
33 Jialal I, Devaraj S. Low density lipoprotein oxidation, antioxidants, and atherosclerosis: A clinical biochemistry perspective. Clin Chem 1996:42, 498–506.
34 Kromhout D. Fatty acids, antioxidants, and coronary heart disease from an epidemiological perspective. Lipids 1999:34 Suppl, S27–S31.
35 Todd S, Woodward M, Tunstall-Pedoe H, Bolton-Smith C. Dietary antioxidant vitamins and fiber in the etiology of cardiovascular disease and all-causes mortality: Results from the Scottish Heart Health Study. Am J Epidemiol 1999:150, 1073–80.
36 McNamara DJ. Relationship between blood and dietary cholesterol. Adv Meat Res 1990:6, 63–87.
37 McNamara DJ. Dietary cholesterol: Effects on lipid metabolism. Curr Opin Lipidol 1990:1, 18–22.
38 McNamara D. Cholesterol intake and plasma cholesterol: an update. J Am Coll Nutr 1997:16, 530–34.
39 McNamara DJ. Dietary cholesterol and the optimal diet for reducing risk of atherosclerosis. Can J Cardiol 1995:11 Suppl G, 123G–6G.
40 Howell WH, McNamara DJ, Tosca MA, Smith BT, Gaines JA. Plasma lipid and lipoprotein responses to dietary fat and cholesterol: A meta-analysis. Am J Clin Nutr 1997:65, 1747–64.
41 Clarke R, Frost C, Collins R, Appleby P, Peto R. Dietary lipids and blood cholesterol: Quantitative meta-analysis of metabolic ward studies. Br Med J 1997:314, 112–17.
42 Hegsted DM, Ausman LM, Johnson JA, Dallal GE. Dietary fat and serum lipids: an evaluation of the experimental data. Am J Clin Nutr 1993:57, 875–83.
43 Hopkins PN. Effects of dietary cholesterol on serum cholesterol: a meta-analysis and review. Am J Clin Nutr 1992:55, 1060–70.
44 Ginsberg HN, Karmally W, Siddiqui M, Holleran S, Tall AR, Rumsey SC, Deckelbaum RJ, Blaner WS, Ramakrishnan R. A dose-response study of the effects of dietary cholesterol on fasting and postprandial lipid and lipoprotein metabolism in healthy young men. Arterioscler Thromb 1994:14, 576–86.
45 Ginsberg HN, Karmally W, Siddiqui M, Holleran S, Tall AR, Blaner WS, Ramakrishnan R. Increases in dietary cholesterol are associated with modest increases in both LDL and HDL cholesterol in healthy young women. Arterioscler Thromb 1995:15, 169–78.
46 Knopp RH, Retzlaff BM, Walden CE, Dowdy AA, Tsunehara CH, Austin MA, Nguyen T. A double-blind, randomized, controlled trial of the effects of two eggs per day in moderately hypercholesterolemic and combined hyperlipidemic subjects taught the NCEP step I diet. J Am Coll Nutr 1997:16, 551–61.
47 Farrell DJ. Enrichment of hen eggs with n-3 long-chain fatty acids and evaluation of enriched eggs in humans. Am J Clin Nutr 1998:68, 538–44.

48 Ferrier LK, Caston LJ, Leeson S, Squires J, Weaver BJ, Holub BJ. Alpha-linolenic acid- and docosahexaenoic acid-enriched eggs from hens fed flaxseed: Influence on blood lipids and platelet phospholipid fatty acids in humans. Am J Clin Nutr 1995:62, 81–6.
49 Blanco-Molina A, Castro G, Martin-Escalante D, Bravo D, Lopez-Miranda J, Castro P, Lopez-Segura F, Fruchart JC, Ordovas JM, Perez-Jimenez F. Effects of different dietary cholesterol concentrations on lipoprotein plasma concentrations and on cholesterol efflux from Fu5AH cells. Am J Clin Nutr 1998:68, 1028–33.
50 Moeller SM, Jacques PF, Blumberg JB. The potential role of dietary xanthophylls in cataract and age-related macular degeneration. J Am Coll Nutr 2000:19, 522S–7S.
51 Handelman GJ, Nightingale ZD, Lichtenstein AH, Schaefer EJ, Blumberg JB. Lutein and zeaxanthin concentrations in plasma after dietary supplementation with egg yolk. Am J Clin Nutr 1999:70, 247–51.
52 Lyle BJ, Mares-Perlman JA, Klein BEK, Klein R, Greger JL. Antioxidant intake and risk of incident age-related nuclear cataracts in the Beaver Dam Eye Study. Am J Epidemiol 1999:149, 801–9.
53 Tees RC, Mohammadi E. The effects of neonatal choline dietary supplementation on adult spatial and configural learning and memory in rats. Dev Psychobiol 1999:35, 226–40.
54 Pyapali GK, Turner DA, Williams CL, Meck WH, Swartzwelder HS. Prenatal dietary choline supplementation decreases the threshold for induction of long-term potentiation in young adult rats. J Neurophysiol 1998:79, 1790–96.
55 Zeisel SH. Choline: Needed for normal development of memory. J Am Coll Nutr 2000:19, 528S–31S.

Dietary cholesterol as a cardiac risk factor: myth or reality? Ed Anthony R Leeds, Juliet Gray.
©2001. Smith-Gordon. Printed in UK.

Discussion

Various aspects

Questioner
What is the panel's explanation for the French paradox?

Professor Mann
Well, the standard explanation for the French paradox, which may or may not be right, has been related to the effect of alcohol and its effect on HDL and perhaps antioxidant nutrients. I think the other possibility is antioxidant nutrients from other sources. I've never seen it explained in terms of dietary cholesterol.

Dr Griffin
I would certainly add into that the nature of the polyunsaturated fatty acids in their diet. The French have n-6, n-3 ratios of 1 to 3 and we're walking around with ratios of anything up to 20 to 1.

Professor Thompson
A South African friend of mine reckons it might be in the wine, but not in the wine that you drink but the wine with which you cook which he finds to be an extremely good antioxidant which prevents peroxidation of cooking fats. So there's another explanation. But basically I think we don't actually know. The French will always be enigmatic to the British.

Questioner
May I add to this French paradox? Is there any truth in the hypothesis that if we eat within 20 minutes when we are tired, without having a rest, everything will turn to fat?

Dr Griffin
Well, with respect to activity, there is quite a marked clinical variation in your intolerance to dietary fat. In Northern Europe we're usually going to sleep at our peak post-prandial lipaemia, whereas the Southern Europeans are actually waking up at that time and are physically active and that may have implications for our ability to clear potential atherogenic remnants from the circulation, and that is largely through an effect of insulin sensitivity of tissue like adipose tissue.

Professor Thompson
With regard to dietary fat to adipose I suppose it depends upon whether you're tired because you've been taking physical exercise or whether you're tired because you've just had a hard day at the office. There is good evidence to suggest that exercise does promote the clearance of triglycerides post-prandially.

Dr Griffin
Yes, I'm of the view that if we all exercised more, we could worry a lot less about our diet. I totally agree.

Cholesterol absorption

Dr McNamara
One of the things that always has fascinated me about cholesterol absorption is that if you feed someone 100 mg of cholesterol, they still absorb around 55%. If you then feed them 200 mg of cholesterol, they still absorb 55%. It's not a situation where that percentage changes when you get to those upper levels. I'm wondering why that percentage stays the same rather than reflecting a mass effect. In other words, if you can absorb 200 mg, why when you're fed 200 mg do you only absorb 100 mg? I have never understood why this happens.

Professor Thompson
Presumably that reflects the kinetics of the process. If the ABC1 transporter is knocked out, cholesterol absorption seems to be unregulated, and a bigger load does not reduce absorption. Whereas most people will absorb proportionally less cholesterol the greater the amount in the diet.

Questioner
Should everyone with high blood cholesterol levels consume plant stanols and sterols or just those with the apoE 4/4 or 3/4 allele?

Professor Thompson
I think that in the context of the primary prevention of coronary disease, when you're managing patients with hypercholesterolaemia, the first step is always to try to get them to modify their diet along conventional lines. Unfortunately, this doesn't always work and certainly in this country studies suggest that only a 2% reduction in serum cholesterol is likely to be achieved by dietary modification. The plant stanol and sterol esters seem to reproducibly achieve something like a 10 to 15% reduction in LDL and this isn't just an effect observable over 3 weeks. Miettinen and colleagues, for example, showed that this effect was maintained for 12 months. This is the primary prevention of coronary disease, this is a great advance in terms of dietary management, obviously coupled with the other aspects of management. I would be interested to know whether people with existing heart disease who are on statins but are unresponsive get a particularly big benefit from using stanol esters. I don't think that means that one should be exclusive in reserving stanol esters for people with the E4 allele. I think that if you give a combination of stanol and statin, you can often get away with a lower dose of statin than you would otherwise have to give because addition of a stanol ester gives you a 10% reduction in LDL whereas doubling the dose of statin only gives you an additional 6% reduction in LDL. This combination therapy could be less expensive.

Professor Mann
The majority of studies of the plant sterol margarines have not provided details of subjects' genes and yet globally there is a cholesterol reduction, so I think one can make the assumption that the vast majority of people in UK, US and New Zealand populations will benefit from plant sterol margarines. There are probably a substantial number of people who could avoid the use of statin drugs if they were instead to use plant sterol margarines, so I think it's really a very exciting development.

Christine Zarember, Dietitian, Epsom General
As plant stanols are obviously so effective in reducing cholesterol absorption, should we now be considering asking the government to make stanol-ester-containing products available on prescription because the retail price at up to £2.50 for 100 g is quite expensive for quite a large group of the patients when up to 25 g of the product per day is needed?

Professor Thompson
It is expensive but I gather that it's expensive stuff to make. Malcolm Law published a meta-analysis in the British Medical Journal earlier this year of all the studies that have been done on plant stanol and sterol ester margarines, and he estimated that if the entire population used them, then the ensuing 10% reduction in total cholesterol would generate a 25% decrease in coronary heart disease within two years. The government has set as one of its targets reducing coronary heart disease by 40% within 10 years. Use of stanol esters would achieve more than half that target in less than 2 years. However I think the likelihood is miniscule that the government would in fact fund it for the population at large.

Statins

Questioner
Does the use of simvastatin and similar compounds reduce the level of cholesterol synthesis so much that you are in danger of running short of steroid hormones?

Professor Thompson
That is a very reasonable question, which was obviously asked in the early days of statin evolution. All the studies that have been done to date so far show a negligible effect. There has been no reduction in the synthesis of steroid hormones that can be considered of any clinical significance, in particular the gonadal hormones and the adrenal hormones; the latter's response to ACTH is not blunted. So I do not think there is anything to worry about on that score.

Questioner
Is there any difference in mechanism of action between atorvastatin and simvastatin?

Professor Thompson
The overall mechanism of action, in other words competitive inhibition of HMG CoA

reductase, is identical. The main difference is that atorvastatin and its metabolites persist in the liver for longer after a single dose than does simvastatin. In other words, its duration of action is longer and that seems to be the reason why it is better at reducing LDL cholesterol than simvastatin.

Questioner
I'm a dietitian working in the field of elderly medicine, advising people over the age of 65. Some reports suggest having a slightly higher cholesterol might be beneficial. Would you like to comment on that?

Professor Thompson
I think there are two things to consider. I think that the importance of cholesterol, particularly LDL cholesterol, as a risk factor becomes less as you get older. I think there's no doubt about that and that by the age of 75, it doesn't matter too much whether you've got a high or an average cholesterol because you've probably got quite advanced vascular disease any way. On the other hand the sub-group analysis of the various statin trials suggests that up to the age of 75 everybody benefits equally from having their LDL reduced by a statin, irrespective of whether they're 60 to 75 or 45 to 60. The relationship between cholesterol as a risk factor and stroke has never been a particularly good one, and yet in the statin trials there was just under a 30% reduction in stroke when cholesterol was reduced. The message is that if you think that someone's going to benefit from having their cholesterol lowered because they've got evidence of vascular disease, then treat them irrespective of their age.

Questioner
The apoE4 polymorphism is associated also nowadays with Alzheimer's disease in the brain, is it not?

Professor Thompson
Yes. In the early onset familial Alzheimer's disease, one of the major risk factors seems to be possession of an apoE4 allele. However, I do not think there is any intention to screen people with a family history of Alzheimer's until there is a means of preventing it.

Other polymorphisms

Questioner
You did not mention at all the apoB and the apoA IV polymorphisms nor indeed some of the others, which are said to determine response to dietary cholesterol. Do you think they are important?

Professor Thompson
No, I do not think they are unimportant but I did not have time to discuss them. I think apoA IV polymorphism may well be involved in cholesterol absorption. I have never been particularly impressed with the data on apoB polymorphisms playing a role, even though apoB is the central protein involved in both chylomicron and LDL formation. It seems to me that MTP is the most important determinant of what happens after cholesterol has actually got into the mucosa, but the biggest unanswered question in this whole field is, what is it that translocates cholesterol across the mucosa? Conceivably, inward movement of cholesterol occurs at a fixed rate and net absorption is largely regulated in the opposite direction, by ABC1. This is a very interesting area of research at present, which could have major therapeutic implications in the future.

Atherogenicity of particles

Professor Thompson
Chris Packard showed that feeding dietary cholesterol resulted in an increase in LDL synthesis, presumably via the VLDL pathway. Is the LDL that's synthesised in response to dietary cholesterol large or small? I would assume it would probably be large.

Dr Griffin
The size of the LDL is very much dependent on the nature and composition of the VLDL that is produced. In normotriglyceridaemic individuals fed cholesterol, the output of VLDL is increased but it's a small, relatively triglyceride-poor VLDL particle which does not lead to small, dense LDL, but probably to LDL in the larger intermediate range. So as in familial hypercholesterolaemia LDL particles of intermediate size are produced.

Professor Thompson
And such particles are less atherogenic unless they are present in large numbers.

Questioner
Has there been any chemical analysis of the plaques removed by surgeons who do endarterectomies? In differentiating roles for cholesterol and triglyceride can chemical analysis throw some light on this particular problem?

Dr Griffin
You don't find triglycerides in plaque to the same extent as cholesterol. You do find oxidised LDL and the sub-fractions of LDL in plaque. The small dense LDL shows increased susceptibility to oxidative modification once it gets into the intima of the arterial wall. It also shows preferential binding to the extracellular tissue matrix. Small dense oxidised LDL particles can be recovered from plaque providing evidence to link an atherogenic lipoprotein phenotype with the atherogenic process.

Professor Thompson
The particular triglyceride-rich lipoproteins that seem to be associated with atherogenesis are the so-called remnant particles, remnants because all the triglyceride has gone, and it's just the cholesterol that's left. It's the cholesterol and not the triglyceride that causes the damage to the artery.

Dr Griffin
I think that it's important to distinguish between the direct effects of triglyceride-rich remnants or remnant particles and the indirect effects of particles that were triglyceride-rich in modulating the structure and properties of LDL and HDL. There are direct and indirect effects of these remnant particles.

Patterns of prescribing and safety of statins

Questioner
Where you showed distributions for levels of prescribing within health authorities for different drugs are the health authorities at the bottom of the distribution the same ones for each distribution?

Dr Ferguson
Very broadly they are the same. The lowest half dozen are in the Greater London area. There are reasons why prescribing may appear lower in the London area, including high rates of registering and de-registering reflecting high levels of population movement. There is always doubt about the population demoninator figures for the London area. Nevertheless across the country as a whole there is (in almost all areas of prescribing) a very clear north-south gradation. Prescribing of everything is lower in the south and higher in the north. It's because there is a more affluent, better-informed population which is more interested in health in the south, and there are more people with chronic illness, fewer resources, more unemployment and more deprivation in the north. Statin prescribing is one of the few areas where the north-south gradation is not seen.

Professor Thompson
I thought that those data were very interesting indeed, particularly the mismatch between need and expenditure. Do you tell the authorities what they are doing and do they know what their CHD rates are? Are they then able to put the two together, relating prescribing to risk?

Dr Ferguson
We feed all this information back to individual prescribers, to community pharmacists, to prescribing advisors in health authorities and so on, and we do quite a large educational programme related to this, to try and make the prescribing patterns better understood.

Professor Thompson
The increase in expenditure on statins with time reflects, I'm sure, the strength of the evidence from trials. You pointed out that fibrate prescribing has stayed stable, probably reflecting a perceived lack of evidence. However, very recent reports of trials, the Veterans Administration HDL intervention trial (VAHIT), and the DAIS trial (fibrate use in diabetic people), demonstrate benefits and expenditure on fibrates may now increase.

Questioner
Dr Ferguson, do you have any figures for the incidence of side-effects from statins?

Dr Ferguson
When a new drug is introduced the side-effects profile of the first ten to twenty thousand patients is monitored. The evidence for statins is in the public domain – the results confirm their safety and low incidence of side-effects.

Professor Thompson
Based on published literature and my own experience of using statins since 1983, I would say that they are incredibly safe, and the frequency of side-effects is much less than for most other drugs.

Plasma homocysteine

Questioner
Dr McNamara, have you looked at your evidence from the point of view of the methionine content of protein foods? It's interesting now to regard protein not just as protein but as a source of cysteine, methionine, arginine etc.

Dr McNamara
The methionine content of eggs is well known. We have asked the question does adding two eggs a day to the diet increase plasma homocysteine levels and the answer is no. So there is no suggestion that eating eggs would increase plasma homocysteine.

Questioner
Is there genetic susceptibility to hyperhomocystinaemia?

Professor Thompson
There's a disease, hyperhomocystinuria, and affected individuals have very high homocysteine levels and this does give rise to very premature coronary disease. There's no doubt that homocysteine is a potential endothelial toxin as animal feeding studies demonstrate endothelial damage. The question is whether it is an endothelial toxin within the range of levels seen in the population at large. I think that we have to wait for the results of the folic acid intervention trials before we can be certain about that.

Questioner
And this would be totally independent of levels of LDL and HDL?

Professor Thompson
It wouldn't change LDL levels at all, but there might be interaction between homocysteine and LDL, in the way that there is, for example, between lipoprotein (a) and LDL. In general terms, I think that the higher your LDL, the more susceptible you are to almost anything else in life in the way of risk factors.

Dr McNamara
And that includes smoking.

Composition of eggs

Questioner
There are reports that genetically modified eggs that are cholesterol free are under development in Australia and in the States. Is that true and has anyone heard about that?

Professor Thompson
Is it possible to achieve that? I think you can perhaps reduce the cholesterol content but to have a cholesterol-free egg I would have thought would be impossible.

Dr McNamara
The attempts to get a low cholesterol egg have really been fraught with difficulty just because of the biological needs of the egg. The primary goal is not to feed us but to develop the chick. The cholesterol is used for embryo development.

Professor Thompson
And low cholesterol eggs?

Dr McNamara
By feeding lovastatin to chickens and the egg cholesterol content can be reduced down to about 140 mg. But for breeding purposes they have to take them off the drug.

Priscilla Marmot
As an Australian dietitian practising in the UK may I comment on the Australian omega-3-enhanced eggs. The cholesterol content of

these eggs has not been altered but the omega-3 fatty acid content is high in relation to omega-6 fatty acids.

Dr McNamara
In Australia omega-3-enhanced eggs are still very popular. Every supermarket has omega-3 eggs for sale at a premium price. I would think that they are beneficial if we believe that there's a risk of very high intakes of omega-6 fatty acids because there are risks of very high risks in several ways, not least of which is oxidation. Omega-3-enhanced eggs may soon be available in the UK but in general terms omega-3-enriched foods are not available in the UK. Britain is also behind the rest of the world in terms of trans fatty acid content of margarines. In Australia and North America, manufacturers have already got rid of trans fatty acids.

Professor Thompson
In fact in the UK it's very easy to get margarines which don't have trans fatty acids (Flora and Benecol contain none) and certainly the latest COMA report recommended that we reduce the content of trans fatty acids in the British diet by at least 50%.

Questioner
I'm a clinical ophthalmologist. I was interested in Dr McNamara's comment about carotenoids and age-related macular degeneration. Could you comment more about that?

Dr McNamara
The carotenoid age-related macular degeneration story is just developing. There has not yet been a good feeding trial to show whether, in people who have the early stages of age-related macular degeneration, intakes of carotenoids alter the risk. There are data that indicate that people with low blood levels of carotenoids are at higher risk. We are actually initiating a study comparing egg-yolk-feeding and spinach intake in people who have initial stages of age-related macular degeneration and increasing their egg or spinach consumption to see whether or not there are any differences in progression of the disease. It is interesting to us that you can increase the lutein level in the egg by altering the feed composition. This is something that you can actually modify in an egg. If you put more marigold extract in the feed, you'll get a much brighter yolk and that yolk has a much higher content of lutein.

Epidemiology

Professor Thompson
In the Health Professionals and Nurses Studies (cited by Dr McNamara) they excluded people with a history of hypercholesterolaemia. They didn't find any relationship between dietary cholesterol and coronary heart disease risk, irrespective of whether they did or did not have hypercholesterolaemia during the study, they didn't actually publish any data on serum lipids in that population. These people were involved in the health business and presumably were a bit more sensible about what they did or didn't do than the public at large. So I suppose you could argue that may be they were a rather selected population and that if you looked at a more representative population sample you might find some sort of relationship between dietary cholesterol and CHD risk.

Dr McNamara
In the Health Professionals and Nurses Studies there was no relationship but in the Mr Fit studies the highest egg consumption was associated with the lowest plasma cholesterol and vice versa. What has never been shown in any study is the association of high plasma cholesterol with high egg consumption.

Dietetic advice

Professor Thompson
Would you give different advice to somebody who has diabetes as far as egg consumption is concerned?

Dr McNamara
I think that at the moment I would recommend that people with diabetes probably maintain the 3 to 4 eggs a week limit. We found no difference in the response of plasma cholesterol to

dietary cholesterol in lean and obese insulin-resistant individuals and in those with normal insulin sensitivity. So insulin-resistance does not seem to influence the effect of dietary cholesterol on plasma cholesterol.

Questioner
Dr McNamara, you've mentioned that for diabetes it's advisable to restrict eggs to about 4 a week, what do you advise for the non-diabetic hyperlipidaemic patient? Are we to assume that it's unlimited or limited to eight that we know won't affect the HDL to LDL ratio?

Dr McNamara
Examination of those 166 cholesterol feeding studies shows that the response of a normocholesterolaemic patient and a hypercholesterolaemic patient is the same, for both LDL and HDL cholesterol. They both go up 1.9 mg/dl for LDL and 0.5 mg/dl for HDL, per 100 mg rise in dietary cholesterol. So there is no indication that a hypercholesterolaemic patient is more sensitive, and there is no indication for restricting egg intake in that population any more than in normocholesterolaemic people.

Dr Keith Ball, retired cardiologist
I was fascinated by your account, Dr McNamara. I'm afraid I came in a minute or so late and I missed the chairman's introduction, and I suppose I'm slightly cynical. I would be concerned if a member of Philip Morris's staff showed that cigarettes really were not harmful and even beneficial, so perhaps you could describe exactly the nature of your association with the egg industry and how any criticisms of bias can be countered.

Dr McNamara
Well my association with the egg industry is that they feed me, they clothe me and they put a roof over my head. Interestingly, I have been a cholesterol researcher since 1966 and actually did some of the first work on HMG CoA reductase, which ended up being a much more interesting enzyme than I thought it was in those early days. I then worked with Peter Irons at Rockefeller University doing clinical studies for 10 years, and then at the University of Arizona doing studies on the effects of dietary cholesterol and dietary fats on lipoprotein metabolism, both in animal models and in patients. In 1995 I was offered the position as Director of the Egg Nutrition Centre which, in the United States, had been in existence at the time for about 14 years and which serves as the health education and research arm of the shell egg industry, overseen by the US Department of Agriculture. We run the health education programme, support roughly a million dollars worth of research each year in Universities and clinical centres around the USA.

The credibility issue comes up a lot and my response is that I present published studies. The evidence I present is found in the Journal of the American Medical Association, the British Medical Journal, the American Journal of Clinical Nutrition and the American Journal of Epidemiology, and I invite anyone who is interested to go and look at those papers and judge the evidence for themselves.

Concluding remarks

Professor Thompson
Dr McNamara has made a convincing case for dietary cholesterol not being a major cause of hypercholesterolaemia or a major contributor to coronary heart disease. Having said that, we live in a country which has one of the highest rates of coronary heart disease in the world. We have very high cholesterol levels which I'm sure is one of the major reasons for that high incidence of coronary heart disease. We have a diet which may be enjoyable but is probably not particularly healthy. And in particular, we still tend to eat our eggs with bacon and we've already agreed that saturated fat as you get it in bacon is not a good idea. So before telling the whole population at large, as well as all our patients, that they can eat as many eggs as they like, we ought to think a little more carefully.

I've spent a lot of time treating patients with familial hypercholesterolaemia and they are usually very good about adhering to dietary advice because they realise that their life may depend upon it. If you tell them, look, you've got to restrict this and that but you don't need to restrict your eggs, they will probably say but aren't eggs very rich in cholesterol? And if you say yes but it doesn't matter having cholesterol in your diet, but it does matter having cholesterol in your blood, I think that one might confuse and give the wrong impression to our patients. So although the scientific data are clear, I think actually trying to transmit that message might be counter-productive. My own feeling is that if somebody knows that they've got a normal cholesterol and they're eating a balanced diet, then I think they should continue to do so, even if their diet happens to contain one or two eggs a day. If they're hypercholesterolaemic, it's conceivable that one reason for the hypercholesterolaemia may be that they are hyper-responders to dietary cholesterol. So I think if they're hypercholesterolaemic, I would be reluctant to tell them that they could eat as many eggs as they like and I feel that one would probably say it would be sensible to keep them to three or four eggs a week.

The other caveat in my mind relates to the effects of plant stanol esters and the way in which one can get a 14% reduction in LDL if one halves cholesterol absorption. This suggests to me that maybe there must be an effect of the amount of dietary cholesterol at the level eaten by most people otherwise it is very difficult to explain the reduction in LDL which occurs when cholesterol absorption is blocked. However it does seem to me that we certainly should be far less stringent about telling people to restrict intake of dietary cholesterol than we have been in the past, although I think we should continue to be very stringent about trying to get them to restrict their intake of saturated fat. Whether we can get both those messages over at the same time without being counter-productive is not clear.

The message then is: if you know that you've a normal cholesterol despite eating eggs, then keep on eating them. If you have a raised cholesterol, then I think you should limit them to two a week.

Dietary cholesterol as a cardiac risk factor: myth or reality? Ed Anthony R Leeds, Juliet Gray.
©2001. Smith-Gordon. Printed in UK.

Index

ABC1 knockout mice 30
Abnormal clotting factors 8, 37
Acyl cholesterol acyl transferase 29
Age as risk factor 7, 63
Age-related macular degeneration 56
Alcohol 36, 61
Alzheimer's disease 63
Antioxidants 55, 61
ApoA 63
ApoB 63
ApoE 8, 22, 30, 32
Atherosclerosis,
    experimental studies and models of 7, 11, 12
    pathology and LDL 17, 61
Atorvastatin 43, 44, 45, 50, 51, 63
ATP-binding cassette transporter 8, 29

Beaver Dam Eye Study 56
Behaviour modification 38
Benecol 32, 52, 66
Bile acids 8, 21–23, 54
Blood glucose as risk factor 8, 36
Body weight 8, 35

Cardiac risk/CHD 7, 12, 35, 36, 38, 53, 54
    and eggs 12, 54
    and general practice 38
Cataract 56
Caveolin 29
Cerivastatin 43–45, 50
Cholestanol 31, 32
Cholesterol
    absorption 8, 17, 21, 27, 29–31, 61, 62
        genetic influences on 17, 29–31, 63
        and LDL 22, 63
    animal studies 9, 12, 54
    biliary excretion 54
    bile acid content of 8, 21–23
    biosynthesis in liver 8, 17, 21
    dietary, adverse, effects of 14, 15
    dietary and atherosclerosis/cardiovascular
        disease
        risk 7, 8, 12, 35–38, 53
        studies of the link between 7, 11, 12, 54–56
    dietary, effects of 17–24, 36, 55
    dietary, epidemiology of 54, 55, 66
        1960–1990 11, 12
    dietary intake levels in research 13, 54, 55
    dietary, and lipids, and metabolism 12–14
    dietary population studies and mortality 11
    dietary, recommendations and restrictions
        7, 14, 15, 20, 53, 61
    dietary and serum/plasma levels 12, 17, 20, 21, 55
        of HDL 19, 56
        of LDL 18, 56, 63
    dietary, and saturated fats 7, 54
    dietary studies and mortality 11
    dietary and tertiles of intake 12
    dietary and triglycerides 24, 63, 64
    egg consumption studies and 13, 14
    feeding studies 7, 12–14, 28, 55, 56, 67
        between 1994–7 20
        eggs and 7, 14, 67
        in animals 11, 12, 28, 30, 54
        in healthy subjects 13, 14, 19, 28
    genetic factors and 7, 38
    hyper-response to 8, 13, 14, 21, 22, 27, 28
    hyporesponse to 14, 20, 21
    hypothesis described 17, 18
    intestinal efflux of 30
    -lowering studies, meta-analysis of 38
    metabolism and homeostasis 41
    response to dietary intake 7, 8, 12–14, 20, 21
        genetic factors 8, 28, 29
        hyper 8, 14, 27, 28
        hypo 8, 14, 27, 28
    serum levels
        dietary intake and 7, 12, 20, 55
        fatty acid intake (s and ps and) and 12, 13
        moderately raised, as risk factor 17
        raised – reduction of and effect on
            coronary mortality 17, 52
    total and reduction by drugs 38
    total – as risk factor 37, 52
    unphysiological levels in studies, 7, 8, 54
Choline 56
Clinical feeding trials 9, 55, 56
Clofibrate 41
COMA
    1984 recommendations 15
    1991 report 20

Index

1994 report 20
Compensatory mechanisms and cholesterol intake 17, 21
Coronary (artery) heart disease 35
  dietary cholesterol and 9
  dietary management 35, 38
  predictors of 12
  risk factors, and management 35, 37
Counselling 8, 38
Counterweight programme 37
Cysteine 65

Diabetes and cholesterol 35, 37, 51, 55
Diet-heart hypothesis 18
Dietary advice 7, 35–38, 67, 68
Dietary fibre 12, 55
Dietitians – role of 35–38, 52

Egg(s)
  cholesterol-feeding studies and 7, 54
  cholesterol high-responders and 8
  clinical feeding trials 55, 56
  composition 65, 66
  consumption 55
    advice on 7, 67
    diabetes and 55, 67
    and heart disease 54, 55
    and mortality rates 55
    national per capita levels 55
    and plasma lipoprotein cholesterol 54, 56, 66
    as proportion of cholesterol intake 14, 54
    recommendations for 9, 53
    restriction and reduction 7, 14, 53–56
    and safety of 56
    and serum LDL 21
  dietary cholesterol and heart disease 54
  epidemiological surveys 54, 55
  nutritional value of 8, 9, 56, 65, 66
  saturated fat content of 54
  US attitudes to 9, 10
  withdrawing from diet: effect of 14
  yolks 28
    cholesterol content of 18
Epidemiological approaches 7, 11, 12, 54, 55, 66
Exercise, role of 7, 35, 61

Familial dyslipidaemias 7, 44, 64
Fatty acids, individual 8, 37
Fibrates, use of 9, 44

Finnish cohort studies 31
Fish oils 8, 37
Flora 66
Fluvastatin 43, 45, 50
Food-based guidelines 38
Framingham Heart Study 54
French paradox, the 61
Functional foods 37, 38

Gender as risk factor 7
General practice
  and cardiac risk 38
  and prescriptions 51
Genetics 8, 29–31
  candidate genes 7, 8, 29
  dietary cholesterol, susceptibility to adverse effects 36
Glucose metabolism, abnormal 36

Health messages 7, 48
  delivery of 48
  need for consistency 52
  scientific basis of 36
Health Professionals Studies 66
Hegsted's formula for dietary cholesterol 13
High-density-lipoprotein 19, 30, 37
  low levels as risk factor 8, 36, 37
  response to dietary cholesterol 19, 20, 30, 56
HMG CoA reductase 14, 32
Homocysteine 65
Honolulu Heart Program 12
Hypercholesterolaemia
  apoE 4 and 8, 31
  management and treatment 8, 41, 44, 62
  pharmacological management in primary care 9, 44, 51
  prescribing and prevention 51, 52
Hyperhomocystinaemia 65
Hyperhomocystinuria 65
Hyperinsulinaemia 37
Hyper-response to cholesterol 13, 14, 21, 22, 28, 56
Hypertension as risk factor 8, 35
Hypertriglyceridaemia as risk factor 8, 36, 37
Hyporesponse to cholesterol 27, 28

Insulin
  levels as risk factor 8, 36
  resistance 8, 38
Ion exchange resins 44
Ireland-Boston Diet Heart Study 12

Keys's formula and equations for dietary cholesterol 12, 13, 18, 20
Keys and Hegsted dietary scores 12

Lathosterol 31
Lifestyle advice 7, 35, 38
Lifestyle change
   counselling to help 37, 38
   importance of 8
   interventions 38
Linoleic acid 14
Linseed oil 41
Lipid-lowering interventions
   advice to patient and 35
   drug prescription and use 44–52
Lovastatin 65
Low-density-lipoprotein cholesterol
   catabolism 20
   egg consumption and 21, 54
   and genetic factors 17, 29–32
   and high-cholesterol feeding 14, 63
   and plant stanol/sterol esters 32, 61
   receptor 7, 18, 22
      as risk factors 65
   saturated fat and 20, 21
   serum levels
      and apoE 22
      and dietary cholesterol 17, 18, 54, 56
LDL – HDL ratio 9, 56, 67

Margarines 32, 52, 56, 62, 66
Methionine 65
Mevalonic acid 32
Mortality
   CHD, and statins 45–49
   cholesterol intake and 11
   and drug prescription patterns 8
   and egg consumption 55

National Health Service, England and Wales (NHS)
   and anti-smoking prescription 52
   prescribing patterns in Authorities of 44–52
NCEP Step diet 30
'Nurses' Health Study' 37, 55, 66
Nutritional advice
   attitudes to 35
   and dietary cholesterol 7
   and saturated fats 7

Obesity
   management 37, 38
   as risk factor 8, 35, 37
   in UK 8, 36, 37
Oliver, Michael 41, 44
Omega-3 fatty acids 8, 65, 66

Pharmacological risk prevention 35
Physical activity 61
Plant stanols and sterol 8, 37, 38, 61
Polyunsaturates 61
Post-prandial lipaemia 8, 36, 61
Pravastatin 43–45, 51
Prescribing of lipid-lowering drugs 41–52
Prevention: primary vs secondary 51, 52

Remnant particles 64
Remnant receptor 52
'Reverse onus' 53
Risk management strategies 35
'Round table' of cardiac risk (Ashwell) 35, 36

Saturated fatty acids, cholesterol and CHD 7, 9, 11, 12, 14, 15, 18, 44, 54
   and genetic predisposition 17
Scandinavian Simvastatin Survival study 31, 44
Scavenger receptor class B type 1 29
Seven Countries Study 12, 17, 18
Simvastatin 31, 32, 43–45, 51, 63
Smoking
   as risk factor 7, 9, 52, 65
   treatment to stop 52
Soya-based products 38
Stanols 32, 40, 62
Statins 44–52, 62, 63
   genetics and 8, 32, 62
   new trials of 65
   prescribing pattern 8, 44–52, 64, 65
Stearic acid and LDL-cholesterol 37
Sterol-regulating binding proteins 18
Stroke, cholesterol and 63
Swedish Obesity Study, 37

Tangier disease 30
Tea, polyphenols and 40
Trans fatty acids 66
Triglycerides
   absorption, and cholesterol feeding 28
   and atherogenic particles 63
   HDL and LDL and 24
   moderately raised levels – risk from 8, 17, 24
   serum, as risk factor 24

United States, dietary cholesterol, egg restriction and 9
Upper abdominal obesity 8

VLDL, dietary cholesterol and 63, 64

Weight management 8, 37

Western Electric study 12

Xanthophylls 56

Zutphen Study, the 12
Zyban 52